Essentials
of
Radiation Biology
and
Protection

Steve Forshier, MEd, RT(R)

DELMAR

THOMSON LEARNING™

Australia Canada Mexico Singapore Spain United Kingdom United States

DELMAR

THOMSON LEARNING

Essentials of Radiation Biology and Protection
by Steve Forshier, MEd, RT(R)

Helath Care Publishing Director:
William Brottmiller

Executive Editor:
Cathy L. Esperti

Acquisitions Editor:
Candice Janco

Developmental Editor:
Darcy M. Scelsi

Editorial Assistant:
Maria D'Angelico

Executive Marketing Manager:
Dawn F. Gerrain

Channel Manager:
Jennifer McAvery

Production Editor:
Mary Colleen Liburdi

Cover Design:
Mary Colleen Liburdi

Library of Congress Cataloging-in-Publication Data on file.

ISBN: 0766813304

NOTICE TO THE READER

Contents

Preface

The purpose of ***Essentials of Radiation Biology and Protection*** is to teach radiologic science students both why and how they can protect themselves and their patients from ionizing radiation. This text will prepare radiography students for the certification examination by the American Registry of Radiologic Technologists (ARRT). This book should also serve as a valuable reference for the practicing radiographer.

This text was born out of a love for teaching the challenging subject of radiation biology and protection to the radiography students at Pima Medical Institute in Mesa, Arizona for the past ten years. Although other texts discuss how to practice radiation protection from a technical viewpoint, this text goes beyond that.

It is vital that we view clinical knowledge and practices as being equally important as theoretical knowledge. This text serves to integrate the theory of radiation protection as seen in radiobiology with radiation protection as it should be practiced in the clinical education setting. Thus, the information presented is both applied and practical for the student and practicing radiographer.

Each chapter begins with an outline, objectives, and key terms and ends with key concepts, review questions, case studies, and recommended reading. The overall design groups the seven chapters into three sections titled:

- Theory and Concepts
- Biological Effects of Radiation Exposure
- Radiation Protection

This design helps organize the content for the student and instructor. Although the ordering of the chapters is based on my experience as a radiography educator, chapters can stand alone and can be used in the order that is most appropriate within a given program.

In addition to the text, ancillary materials include an instructor's manual and a student workbook. The instructor's manual contains self-assessment questions with answers, case studies with answers, and a test bank of questions with answers. The student workbook includes questions and case studies that are different from the ones found in the instructor's manual.

Although I assume full responsibility for any errors, including those that may be construed as arising from quoting other works out of context, I have made every effort to ensure the accuracy of the information. Neither the author nor the publisher takes responsibility or accepts any liability for the actions of persons applying the information contained herein in an unprofessional manner. This information is designed to supplement and enhance the instructional methodologies of educators in Joint Review Committee on Education in Radiologic Technologists (JRCERT) approved radiography program, and should not be applied, especially to human subjects, without this background. While committing this book to print, I realize that it is never really completed, but is merely a work in progress.

References used extensively to assure both educator and students that we address all content expected for successful professional practice include the American Registry of Radiographic Technologists' (ARRT) *Content Specifications for the Examination in Radiography*, and the American Society of Radiologic Technologists' (ASRT) *Curriculum Guide for Radiography Programs.*

No text is created without the assistance of many individuals whose names do not appear on the title page. This book is no exception. I would like to express my sincere appreciation and gratitude to the following individuals who contributed significantly to this project.

First and foremost to my best friend, my wife Pam, who has always supported my endeavors.

To all the staff at Delmar Thomson Learning, especially to Darcy Scelsi, Developmental Editor, for her endless support and contributions.

To the reviewers of this text, their contributions helped to improve the text significantly.

Theory and Concepts

CHAPTER 1 *History of Radiobiology*

CHAPTER 2 *Cellular Anatomy and Physiology*

CHAPTER 3 *Cellular Effects of Radiation*

Radiobiology may be defined as the branch of science concerned with the methods of interaction and the effects of ionizing radiation on living systems. It is a combination of biology, physics, and epidemiology. Since many radiation effects take place at the cellular level, those people who deal with ionizing radiation should have an understanding of cell structure and function, and how these can be affected by exposure to ionizing radiation. This section focuses on the theory and concepts of radiobiology.

History of Radiobiology

OBJECTIVES

Upon completion of this chapter, the reader should be able to:

- Discuss the history of radiobiology
- Identify leaders in the field of radiobiology and their contributions to research
- Define terms related to the measurement of radiation
- Identify regulations related to the field of radiobiology

RADIOBIOLOGY HISTORY

Three incidents triggered the beginning of radiobiology: Wilhelm Conrad Roentgen's discovery of x-rays in 1895; Henri Becquerel's observance of rays being given off by a uranium-containing substance in 1896 (Marie Curie subsequently would call this **radioactivity**); the discovery of radium by Pierre and Marie Curie in 1898.

Early radiobiology observations included skin **erythema** (radiation induced skin reddening), **epilation** (radiation induced hair loss), and **anemia**. Because of unshielded fluoroscopic apparatus, radiologists had to have fingers amputated, and compared with other doctors, had elevated incidence of leukemia.

The first United States x-ray fatality occurred in 1906. Clarence Daly, an assistant of Thomas Edison, had collaborated with him in producing the fluoroscope and fluorescent screens. In working long days, Daly was subjected to doses above modern lifetime limits. In Edison's day, shielding was seldom used for personnel or x-ray tubes.

The early observations of Becquerel, the Curies, and early radiologists sparked much research into the effects of radiation exposure on biological processes. Beginning in the early 1900s through the 1950s and 1960s, many theories were developed to define and explain these effects.

Law of Bergonie and Tribondeau

In 1906 two Frenchmen, J. Bergonie and L. Tribondeau, exposed rodent testicles to x-rays, and observed the effects of radiation. They selected the testes since this organ contains both mature cells (spermatozoa), which execute the organ's principal function, and immature cells (spermatogonia and spermatocytes), whose only purpose is to evolve into mature, functional cells. Not only do these cells' functions differ, but their rate of mitosis (see Chapter 2) also differs. The spermatogonia (immature) cells divide frequently, whereas the spermatozoa (mature) cells do not divide. After exposing the testes to radiation, Bergonie and Tribondeau noticed that the immature cells were injured at doses lower than the mature cells. Supported by these observations, they proposed a law describing the radiation sensitivity for all body cells. Their law maintains that actively mitotic and undifferentiated cells are most susceptible to damage from ionizing radiation.

The **law of Bergonie and Tribondeau** states that:

1. Stem cells are more radiosensitive than mature cells. The more mature a cell is, the more radioresistant.
2. Younger tissues and organs are more radiosensitive than older tissues and organs.
3. The higher the metabolic activity of a cell, the more radiosensitive it is.
4. The greater the proliferation and growth rate for tissues, the greater the radiosensitivity.

This law informs us that compared to a child or mature adult, the fetus is most radiosensitive.

Ancel and Vitemberger

In 1925 the law of Bergonie and Tribondeau was modified by P. Ancel and P. Vitemberger. They suggested that the intrinsic susceptibility of damage to any cell by ionizing radiation is the same, but that the timing of manifestation of radiation-produced damage varies according to the types of cells. In experiments on mammals, they determined that there are two factors which affect the appearance of radiation damage to the cell:

1. The amount of biologic stress the cell receives.
2. Pre- and post-irradiation conditions that the cell is exposed to.

Ancel and Vitemberger theorized that the most significant biologic stress on the cell is the need for division. In their terms, a given dose of radiation will cause the same degree of damage to all cells (the innate susceptibility is comparable for all cells) but only if and when the cell divides will damage be demonstrated.

Even though Ancel and Vitemberger communicate radiosensitivity differently than Bergonie and Tribondeau, they do agree with them by placing a significant emphasis on the amount of mitotic activity involved.

In the 1920s researchers learned that the process of ionization in tissues was the cause of biologic results. The two mechanisms recognized were:

- Direct ionization along charged particle tracks caused **direct effects** (original ionization occurs directly on target molecule)
- The formation of free radicals caused **indirect effects** (original ionization occurs with water, and transfers ionization to target molecule).

Fractionation Theory

The 1920s and 1930s brought the **fractionation** theory from France. Ram testicles were exposed to large doses of ionizing radiation. Even though the rams could be sterilized with one large dose, this quantity of radiation also caused the skin adjacent to the ram's scrotum to have a reaction. It was found, however, that if the large dose was fractionated (smaller doses spread out over a period of time), the animals would still become sterile, but with considerably less damage to their skin.

Mutagenesis

In 1927 H. Muller discovered that ionizing radiation produced mutations through his experiments with fruit flies. His finding is termed **mutagenesis**. He found that the radiation-induced mutations were the same as those produced in nature. Irradiating the fruit flies did not create any unusual effects, but the frequency of mutations was intensified. This implies that the effects of ionization were not unique to radiation, that is, they could have been caused by things other than radiation.

Effects of Oxygen

The oxygen effect was the subject of experimentation during the 1940s and 1950s. Oxygen is termed a radiosensitizer because it increases the cell-killing effect of a given dose of radiation. This occurs as a result of the increased production of free radicals when ionizing radiation is delivered in the presence of oxygen.

Reproductive Failure

In 1956, Puck and Marcus exposed human uterine cervix cells to varying doses of radiation. They experimentally determined **reproductive failure** by counting the number of colonies formed by these irradiated cells.

As scientists began to research the effects that radiation exposure had on biological processes, there arose a need to measure the levels of radiation causing specific effects. Units of measurement were developed to quantify radiation levels and thus track the effects of exposure by varying the levels of exposure.

Roentgen

1928 saw the creation of the term **roentgen** (R). It was defined as a unit of radiation quantity. The roentgen is a measure of the ionization of air that is created by x- and gamma-radiation below 3 MeV (3 million electron volts). X-ray machine outputs are specified in roentgens or milliroentgens (mR). The adoption of the Roentgen as a unit of measurement created the basic tool for defining standards of protection for personnel. In 1937 the roentgen was internationally accepted, and is defined as 1 R = 2.58 x 10^{-4} coulomb/kg air.

Rad

The **rad** (an acronym for radiation absorbed dose) was officially adopted in 1953, and equals the absorption of 10^{-2} J of energy per kilogram (or 100 ergs/g) of absorbing material.

$$1 \text{ rad} = 10^{-2} \text{ J/kg} = 100 \text{ ergs/g}$$

The rad describes the energy that is absorbed in matter from any type of ionizing radiation, and is considered the unit of absorbed dose.

Rem

The **rem** (an acronym for radiation equivalent man) is the unit of dose equivalent (DE) or occupational exposure. The rem represents the amount of radiation received by personnel. The rem is said to have approximately the same biologic effectiveness as 1 rad of x-ray. Thus, 1 R = 1 rad = 1 rem in diagnostic radiology.

SI Units

In 1948, the International Committee for Weights and Measures developed a system of measurement that was meant to standardize units of measurement; this unit of measurement is known as the System Internationale d'Unites or SI units. Within this system of measurement the traditional units of rotengen, rad, and rem are no longer applicable. Exposure is now measured by coulomb per kilogram, as the unit of measure replacing the rotengen. Absorbed dose is now expressed by the gray (Gy), which replaces the rad. One gray is equivalent to 100 rads. The equivalent dose is now expressed by the sievert; formerly known as the rem. Although the National Council on Radiation Protection and Measurement adopted the use of SI units in 1985, traditional units are still in use. The radiologist should have a working knowledge of both traditional and SI units. Table 1–1 presents the conversion of traditional units to SI units. Table 1–2 compares both the SI and traditional units.

REGULATION

There are many different organizations and agencies that are responsible for the development of standards and regulations for radiation protection. Some of these groups include the International Commission of Radiological Protection (ICRP) formed in 1928; and in the United States, the National Council on Radiation Protection and Measurement (NCRP) chartered by Congress in 1964, the Nuclear Regulatory Commission (NRC), and the Food and Drug Administration (FDA).

The International Commission of Radiological Protection and the organization now known as the National Council on Radiation Protection and Measurement first began promoting the idea of regulating the amount

TABLE 1–1

CONVERSIONS BETWEEN CONVENTIONAL AND SI UNITS		
Conventional Unit (Column A)	**Conversion Factor (Column B)**	**SI Unit (Column C)**
roentgen	2.58×10^4	coulomb/kilogram
rad	0.01	gray
rem	0.01	sievert
curie	3.7×10^{10}	becquerel

Column A amount multiplied by Column B equals Column C amount.
Column C amount divided by Column B equals Column A amount.

(From Carlton, R., & Adler, A. [2001]. *Principles of radiographic imaging: An art and science* [3rd ed.]. Albany, NY: Delmar/Thomson Learning.

TABLE 1–2

COMPARISON BETWEEN SI AND CONVENTIONAL UNITS

Quantity	Symbol for Quantity	Expression in SI Units	Expression in Symbols for SI Units	Special Name for SI Units	Symbol Using Special Name	Conventional Unit	Symbol for Conventional Unit	Value of Conventional Unit in SI Units
Activity	A	1 per second	s^{-1}	becquerel	Bq	curie	Ci	3.7×10^{10} Bq
Absorbed Dose	D	joule per kilogram	J/kg	gray	Gy	rad	rad	0.01 Gy
Dose Equivalent	H	joule per kilogram	J/kg	sievert	SV	rem	rem	0.01 Sv
Exposure	X	coulomb per kilogram	C/kg			roentgen	R	2.58×10^{-4} C/kg

(From Carlton, R., & Adler, A. [2001]. *Principles of radiographic imaging: An art and science* [3rd ed.]. Albany, NY: Delmar/Thomson Learning.

of exposure for personnel in the field of radiography in 1931. Based upon the research of these two organizations the recommended permissible dose was set at 0.2R/day. In 1962 the personnel maximum permissible dose (MPD), now known as dose-equivalent limit, was set at 5 rem/yr.

In 1977 the International Council on Radiation Protection (ICRP) Publication 26 set an annual occupational exposure limit of 5 rem per year, and the dose limit for the public of 500 mrem (0.5 rem) per year. In 1991 the ICRP further reduced the occupational exposure limit to 2 rem per year. This recommendation is not yet being enforced in the United States.

In January 1994 the Nuclear Regulatory Commission (NRC) set dose equivalent limits based on the National Council on Radiation Protection (NCRP) Report No. 91, which has limits of 5 rem per year for occupational exposure, and 0.1 rem for frequent exposure per year for the public. The public is allowed 0.5 rem annually for infrequent exposure. The differences between the new 10CFR20 and the old are outlined in Table 1–3.

KEY CONCEPTS

- Wilhelm Conrad Roentgen is credited with founding the field of radiobiology with his discovery of x-rays. Much research was done in the 1920s on the effects of radiation on biological processes. Today research continues on the effects of low level radiation in exposed workers.

TABLE 1–3

COMPARISON OF REQUIREMENTS OF OLD NRC REGULATION 10CFR20 TO NEW NRC REGULATION 10CFR20

	Old 10CFR20	New 10CFR20
Whole body definition	Head, lens of eyes, trunk, gonads, arms above elbow, legs above ankle	Head, trunk, gonads, arms above elbow, legs above knee
Extremities definition	Arms elbows and below, legs ankle and below	Arms elbows and below, legs ankle and below
Whole body exposure limits	1.25 rem/calendar quarter **with** maximum 3 rem/qtr **and** 12 rem/yr **if** 5(N-18) not exceeded Note: 5(N-18) is no longer used	Most limiting of: 500 mSv (50 rem)/yr to any organ **or** 50 mSv (5 rem)/yr whole body
Lens of the eye	1.25 rem/qtr, maximum 3 rem/qtr and 12 rem/yr if 5(N-18) not exceeded	150 MsV (15 rem)/yr
Skin of the whole body	7.5 rem/qtr and 30 rem/yr	500 MsV (50 rem)/yr
Extremities	18.75 rem/qtr and 75 rem/yr applied to any part of any extremity	500 MsV (50 rem)/yr applied to each extremity
Embryo/fetus/pregnancy		5 mSv/term (0.5 rem or 500 mrem)

(From Carlton, R., & Adler, A. [2001]. *Principles of radiographic imaging: An art and science* [3rd ed.]. Albany, NY: Delmar/Thomson Learning.

- Bergonie and Tribondeau theorized that younger, immature tissues and organs are more radiosensitive than older tissues and organs. They also discovered that the more metabolic activity within a cell the more radiosensitive the cell was. Ancel and Vitemberger determined that radiation damage is determined by the amount of biological stress the cell receives and the conditions the cell is exposed to before and after radiation. Muller made the discovery of radiation's role in mutation termed mutagenesis.
- The roentgen is a unit of radiation quantity (1 R = 2.58×10^{-4} coulomb/kg). Rad measures the energy absorbed in matter from any type of radiation (1 rad = 10^{-2} J/kg = 100 ergs/g). Rem is the unit of dose equivalent or occupational exposure.
- 5 rem per year is the maximum permissible dose for occupational exposure. 0.1 rem is the limit for frequent public exposure and 0.5 rem is the limit for infrequent public exposure.

Cellular Anatomy and Physiology

KEY TERMS

Amino acid

Anabolism

Anaphase

Autosome

Catabolism

Centromere

Chromatid

Chromatin

Chromosome

Deoxyribonucleic acid (DNA)

Diploid

Duplication

Enzyme

G_1

G_2

Gamete

Gene

Haploid

Interphase

Macromolecule

Meiosis

Messenger RNA

Metaphase

Mitosis

Nuclear membrane

Nuclear membrane

Nucleolus

Organism

Polymer

Prophase

Protoplasm

Ribonucleic acid (RNA)

Ribosomal RNA

S-phase

Telophase

Transfer RNA

OBJECTIVES

Upon completion of this chapter, the reader should be able to:

- Indicate the parts of the cell
- Identify organic compounds and their functions
- Identify inorganic compounds and their functions
- Explain mitosis
- Explain meiosis

CELL BIOILOGY

In order to appreciate radiation interactions within cells, a review of cell biology is necessary. All living things, whether plant or animal, are made up of cells. The cell is the basic unit of structure and function of all living things. It is at the cellular level that the fundamental life functions occur. These essential functions include metabolism, growth, irritability, adaptability, repair, and reproduction. All cells are made up of chemical material called **protoplasm**. The cell is the smallest unit of protoplasm capable of existing independently.

Humans contain between 60 and 100 trillion cells. These cells vary in size, shape, and function. With the exception of human ovum or egg cells, human cells are microscopic in size. They are measured in units called micrometers (μm), or microns (μ) (1 μm or μ = 1/1,000,000 or 0.000001 or 10^{-6} or approximately 1/25,000 of an inch). These units of measurement are used when describing cell sizes and their cell components.

Regarding shape, human cells differ tremendously. Their shapes may be spherical, rectangular, or irregular. The human body has numerous distinct types of cells, each of which is specialized in performing particular functions. Bone cells, muscle cells, fat cells, blood cells, and nerve cells are examples of specialized cells. Cell structure is directly related to its function.

Tissues are collections of similar cells that work together in performing a particular function. An example of a tissue is muscle. Muscles function to contract and cause movement of body parts.

An organ is a combination of two or more tissues that are combined to perform a specific function. Organs vary greatly in their size and function. The heart, spleen, and pancreas are examples of organs.

The system is the next level of structural organization. Organs that have similar or related functions comprise a body system. The digestive system and circulatory system are examples of systems. All the body systems work together and are interrelated to form the total organism.

Chemical Configuration of Cells

Protoplasm contains organic and inorganic compounds. These are either dissolved or suspended in water, which is the most abundant component of protoplasm. Protoplasm contains 70–85% water. The percentage of water in protoplasm depends upon the type of cell. Water makes up approximately 55–75% of a person's total body weight, and for several reasons is essential to life. The critical functions of water in the body include:

- qction as a solvent, that is, various substances can dissolve in water
- acts as a transport medium for substances
- serves to lubricate joints and the digestive tract
- regulates body temperature through evaporation
- cushions organs such as the brain and lungs

Organic Compounds   Organic compounds denote chemical substances which contain carbon. The four major classes of organic compounds found in cells include proteins, carbohydrates, nucleic acids, and lipids.

Proteins   Proteins, which comprise 15% of the cell, are composed of the elements carbon, hydrogen, oxygen, and nitrogen. Proteins are found in all parts of a living cell. Functions of proteins include: assisting in growth, constructing new tissues, and repairing injured or worn-out tissues. Enormous amounts of proteins are located in fingernails, hair, cartilage, ligaments, tendons, and muscle.

Amino acids are the building blocks of proteins. In humans there are 22 different amino acids that combine in numerous sequences to create proteins. The number of amino acids in proteins ranges from 300 to several thousand. Examples of proteins include insulin, egg whites, gelatin, and hemoglobin.

Enzymes are an important group of proteins that are found in all living cells. Enzymes act as organic catalysts. They control the numerous chemical reactions that occur in cells. Enzymes provide cell energy, help to make new cell parts, and control almost every cell process. They affect the rate or speed of chemical reactions without themselves being altered.

Lipids   Lipids comprise approximately 2% of the cell. Lipids contain carbon, hydrogen, and oxygen, and exist in all living cells. Lipids function in storing energy, insulating our bodies from cold, assisting with the digestive process, and helping to lubricate the joints.

Carbohydrates   Carbohydrates make up approximately 1% of the cell. They are composed of carbon, hydrogen, and oxygen, and are the major source of cell energy. Even though carbohydrates are found throughout the body, they are located predominately in the liver and muscles. Carbohydrates are subdivided into: monosaccharides, disaccharides, and polysaccharides. Monosaccharides are considered simple sugars. They cannot be broken down further. Examples are glucose, fructose, and galactose. Disaccharides are known as double sugars. Examples include sucrose (table sugar), and lactose (milk sugar). Polysaccharides are large **macromolecules** constructed of hundreds to thousands of simple sugar molecules in a long chain. Examples include starch and cellulose.

Nucleic Acids   Nucleic acids are organic compounds that contain carbon, oxygen, hydrogen, and phosphorus. They are the largest known organic molecules. Nucleic acids are high-molecular-weight **polymers** made from thousands of smaller subunits called nucleotides. Nucleotides are composed of a five-carbon sugar (pentose sugar), a phosphate or phosphoric acid group, and one of many nitrogenous bases. There are two groups of nitrogenous bases, purines and pyrimidines. Purines are either adenine (A) or guanine (G). The pyrimidines are cytosine (C), thymine (T), or uracil (U).

The nucleic acids include **DNA (deoxyribonucleic acid)** and **RNA (ribonucleic acid)**.

Inorganic Compounds   Mineral salts, the inorganic substance in the cell, are essential for cell life. Sodium (Na) and potassium (K) are examples of salts. Potassium inside the cell prevents the cell from collapsing. Sodium outside the cell prevents the cell from bursting. Sodium and potassium maintain the osmotic pressure of the cell by maintaining the correct proportion of water in the cell. Salts are required in order for the cell to function correctly. For example, if there were a deficiency of calcium salts in the cell, muscle cramps would occur. Salts also assist in producing cell energy, and in conducting nerve impulses.

Cell Structure

Even though human cells can be very different, they also have many similar structural characteristics: a cell membrane, cytoplasm and organelles. With the exception of mature red blood cells, all human cells have a nucleus. The cytoplasm, organelles, and nucleus are enclosed by a cell membrane. An diagram of a cell's structure is shown in Figure 2–1.

Cell Membrane   All human cells are surrounded by cell membranes, sometimes called plasma membranes. A cell membrane functions to separate the cell's interior from its exterior surroundings, and also from adjacent cells. Although it is the outer boundary of the cell, a cell membrane is not static, but instead is active and dynamic. Cell membranes are composed of lipids and proteins which are arranged in a double layer, somewhat comparable to a sandwich: the two protein layers are the slices of bread, and the lipids are the filling (Figure 2–2). The cell membrane is considered to be selectively semi-permeable. It allows some substances to pass into and out of the cell, while preventing the passing of others. Lipids allow lipid-soluble materials to diffuse into or out of the cell. Proteins function as pores, enzymes, or antigens.

Cytoplasm   Cytoplasm, composed of proteins, lipids, carbohydrates, minerals, salts, and water, is a watery solution found between the nucleus and cell membrane. Chemical reactions, such as protein synthesis and cellular respiration, take place in the cytoplasm. **Catabolism** (the process of converting a complex substance into a simpler substance) and **anabolism** (the building up of a body's substance) take place in the cytoplasm. Metabolism is the combination of catabolism and anabolism.

Organelles   Cell organelles, located within the cytoplasm, help with cell functioning. Cell organelles include the centrioles, endoplasmic reticulum, mitochondria, Golgi apparatus, lysosomes, and the nucleus.

The Centrosome and Centrioles   The centrioles, a pair of cylindrical organelles located near the nucleus, are perpendicular to each other, and function to organize the spindle fibers during cell mitosis. They are contained in a circular body named the centrosome. During mitosis, the

FIGURE 2–1
Cell structure

pair of centrioles detach from each other. During this detachment, thin cytoplasmic spindle fibers are formed between the centrioles. This formation is known as the spindle-fiber apparatus. Spindle fibers connect to specific chromosomes to aid with the equal disbursement of these chromosomes to two daughter cells.

The Endoplasmic Reticulum   The endoplasmic reticulum (ER) is a tubular network that extends from the nuclear membrane to the cell membrane. The endoplasmic reticulum assists in channeling proteins and lipids into and out of the nucleus. Some ER collects copious amounts of

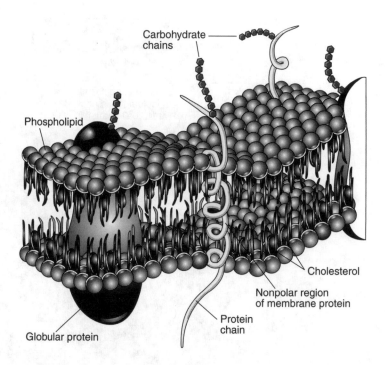

FIGURE 2–2

Plasma membrane

proteins and thus serves as storage areas. The two types of ER are rough and smooth. Rough ER has numerous ribosomes attached to its outer surface, giving it a rough appearance. It is found in cells that are active secretors of proteins, such as the endocrine and exocrine glands. Smooth ER has no ribosomes attached to it. It is a site for enzyme reactions in steroid hormone production and inactivation, and is the part of the cell where many drugs are inactivated. It also serves in storing Ca^{++} in skeletal muscle cells.

The Mitochondria Mitochondria are double-membraned, oval or rod-shaped organelles found in the cytoplasm. The shape and number of mitochondria vary from one cell to another. Aerobic (oxygen-requiring) reactions of cell respiration take place within the mitochondria. The double-membrane of the mitochondria contains enzymes, which assist in breaking down carbohydrates, fat, and proteins into energy, stored in the cell as ATP (adenosine-triphosphate). Cells that require large amounts of ATP contain the greatest amount of mitochondria, such as muscle cells. Because mito-chondria supply the cell's energy; they are nicknamed the "powerhouses" of the cell.

The Golgi Apparatus The Golgi apparatus, also called Golgi bodies or the Golgi complex, was discovered in 1898 by the Italian scientist Camillo Golgi. It is a series of flat, membranous layers, looking somewhat like a stack of pancakes or saucers. Synthesized within the Golgi apparatus are carbohydrates. These carbohydrates are combined with proteins as they pass through the Golgi apparatus, and are concentrated and packaged for secretion from the cell. In order to secrete a substance, small portions of the Golgi membrane separate and join with the cell membrane, which allows the substance to be released to the cell's exterior. These organelles are most abundant in the gastric gland cells, salivary glands, and pancreatic glands.

Lysosomes Lysosomes are single-membrane oval or spherical bodies within the cytoplasm which contain digestive enzymes that digest protein molecules. Lysosomes assist in digesting old, worn-out cell parts, dead cells, bacteria and foreign materials. If a lysosome happens to burst, it begins to digest the cell's protein, causing cell death. This is how they acquired the nickname "suicide bags."

The Nucleus The most vital cell organelle is the nucleus. The nucleus is the brain for the cell's metabolic activity and cell division. Spherical in shape, it is usually located in or near the cell's center. The nucleus floats within the cytoplasm, and is surrounded by a double-layered nuclear membrane. DNA (deoxyribonucleic acid) and protein are contained within the nucleus. DNA and protein are arranged in long threads called **chromatin**. When a cell divides, the chromatin contracts into short, rodlike structures called **chromosomes**. Humans normally have 46 total chromosomes, or 23 pairs.

When particular cells reach certain sizes, they may divide into two new cells. If this occurs, the nucleus divides first by undergoing a process called **mitosis**. During mitosis, nuclear substances are distributed to each new nucleus. Next, the cytoplasm divides approximately in half through the development of a new membrane between the two nuclei. It is exclusively during this process of the nucleus dividing that the chromosomes are visible.

Chromosomes contain the human hereditary blueprint—DNA—which passes from one generation of cells to the next.

The Nuclear Membrane The **nuclear membrane** is double-layered, and has openings through which substances can travel either from the cytoplasm to the nucleus, or from the nucleus to the cytoplasm. The nuclear membrane's outer layer is contiguous with the ER of the cytoplasm, and contains ribosomes. Surrounding the chromatin and nucleoli is the transparent semi-fluid nucleoplasm.

The Nucleolus and Ribosomes Each nucleus contains at least one nucleolus. The tiny, spherical-shaped **nucleolus** contains ribosomes composed of RNA and protein. Ribosomes can travel from the cell's nucleus into the cytoplasm. It is there that ribosomes assist in protein synthesis. Ribosomes exist as single units in the cytoplasm, as clusters called polyribosomes, or joined to the walls of the ER.

DNA and RNA The DNA nucleotide structure is composed of a phosphate group, a deoxyribose sugar, and the nitrogenous bases adenine, thymine, cytosine, and guanine. The RNA nucleotide consists of a phosphate group, ribose sugar, and the nitrogenous bases adenine, cytosine, guanine, and uracil instead of thymine.

The structure of DNA looks like a coiled ladder, as seen in Figure 2–3 The two strands of nucleotides are labeled a double helix (coil). The sides of the ladder are formed by the alternating phosphate and sugar molecules. The rungs of the ladder are formed by the pairs of nitrogenous bases. With DNA, adenine always pairs with thymine, and guanine always pairs with cytosine. An acrostic to help you remember these pairings is At The Grand Canyon. It is estimated that the DNA of our 46 chromosomes includes approximately 6 billion base pairs, which compose from 50,000 to 100,000 genes.

Unique genetic information is carried by the DNA located in the nuclear chromosomes and genes. This genetic material instructs the cell as to what structures it will have, and how it will function and behave. The DNA passes genetic information from cell to cell, and ultimately from generation to generation. Thus, DNA is considered the genetic code for heredity characteristics. DNA is located in the plasma membrane, mitochondria, and centrioles.

Instead of being double-stranded like DNA, RNA is a single-stranded nucleotide, with uracil pairing with adenine in place of thymine. RNA is produced from DNA in the cell nucleus, but functions in the cell's cytoplasm.

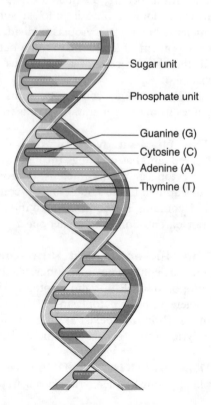

Sugar unit

Phosphate unit

Guanine (G)
Cytosine (C)
Adenine (A)
Thymine (T)

FIGURE 2–3
DNA structure

There are three varieties of RNA. These include **messenger RNA** (m-RNA), **transfer RNA** (t-RNA), and **ribosomal RNA** (r-RNA). Messenger RNA carries directions for protein synthesis from the DNA molecule situated in the cell's nucleus into the cytoplasm, and also carries the code for specific protein synthesis from the DNA in the nucleus to the ribosomes in the cytoplasm. Transfer RNA carries amino acid molecules from the cytoplasm to the ribosomes for protein synthesis. Ribosomal RNA assists in the linking of the messenger RNA to the ribosome. RNA is found in the nucleoli, cytoplasm, and some cell ribosomes.

Chromosomes and Genes Within the nucleus is the substance responsible for guiding the activity of the cytoplasm. This genetic material is enclosed in chromosomes. Chromosomes are only visible in cells that are dividing. The parts of the chromosome include a **centromere**, which is the center of a chromosome, and arms which extend in each direction from the centromere (see Figure 2–4).

The chromosomes carry **genes**, the genetic material responsible for cytoplasmic activity and delivering the cell's hereditary information. Each chromosome contains numerous genes which are situated on the chromosome

Human chromosomes

Supercoil within chromosome

Chromatin

Coiling within supercoil

Chromatin fiber

FIGURE 2–4
Chromosome structure

in a unique linear order. All genes execute specific functions in preserving an organism's life and development.

Sexually reproducing cells in animals are classified as either germ cells or somatic cells. Germ cells are **gametes**: female gametes are termed oocytes, male gametes are called spermatozoa. The somatic cells are all the other cells in the body.

Somatic cells have at least two of each kind of gene situated on two different chromosomes. These two chromosomes are identical in the arrangement and type of genes they carry and are called homologues. Consequently, the chromosomes in somatic cells are paired. Each member of a pair is identical, but the pairs themselves are not alike.

The normal number of chromosomes for humans is 46. This number is termed the **diploid** number, or 2n.

In germ cells, chromosomes and genes are not paired, but are individual chromosomes. These individual chromosomes come from each of the pairs that exist in the somatic cells. Thus, germ cells contain one-half the number of chromosomes and genes present in somatic cells. The number of chromosomes in germ cells is referred to as the **haploid** or n number.

In humans, the somatic cells contain 46 chromosomes in the nucleus, of which 44 are **autosomes** (nonsex chromosomes), and two are sex chromosomes.

In a human female, somatic cells contain 44 autosomes and two sex chromosomes (both are X chromosomes). In the human male, there are also 44 autosomes and two sex chromosomes (an X and a Y chromosome).

The human germ cells have one specific function, which is to reproduce the species. During fertilization, the sperm nucleus unites with the egg nucleus to form a fertilized egg, or zygote. Accordingly, it is essential that each germ cell contain only one-half the number of chromosomes to produce a normal zygote which contains the required 2n number of chromosomes (Figure 2–5).

CELL GROWTH AND DIVISION

Cell life follows a cyclical pattern. A new cell is produced as part of its parent cell. When this daughter cell divides, it becomes two new cells. As long as a cell's offspring continue to divide, each cell is conceivably immortal. Some body cells divide constantly; for example, about every 2–3 days the stomach lining is renewed, and the skin's epidermis is renewed about every two weeks. Conversely, some cells, such as mature nerve cells and skeletal muscle, do not go through division at all.

The two types of cell division are **mitosis** and **meiosis**. Even though both types include reproduction of the cell, their purposes are not similar.

Mitosis

Cell division or mitosis can be divided into two discrete processes: the dividing of the nucleus, and the dividing of the cytoplasm.

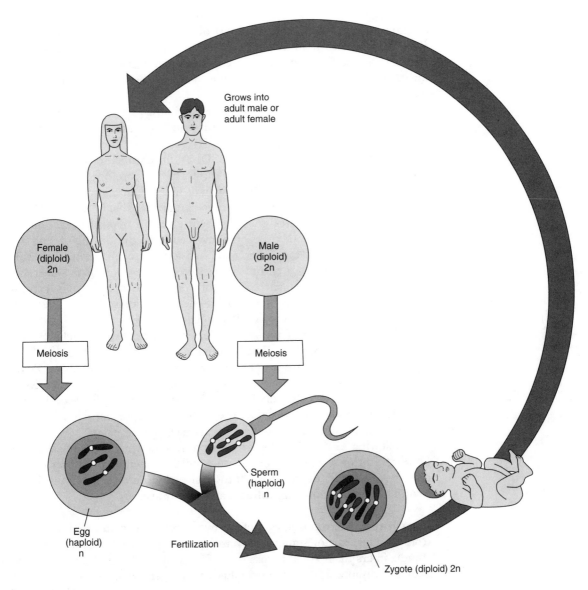

FIGURE 2–5
Diploid and haploid interaction

All human life begins as a fertilized egg. In mitosis, a cell with the diploid number of chromosomes (normally 46) divides into two identical cells, each containing the diploid number of chromosomes. In order for there to be growth of the body and tissue repair, the production of identical cells is essential.

The nondividing cell is in the segment of the cell cycle known as **interphase**, which is subdivided into G_1, S, and G_2. Genes control the metabolism of the cell through their direction of RNA synthesis. Since the cell may be growing during this time, this part of interphase is called the G_1 phase (G = gap or growth). Sometimes referred to as the resting phase, cells in the G_1 phase are performing the physiological purposes necessary to maintaining cell homeostasis. Resting means the cell is not yet undergoing the visible phases of mitosis.

If a cell is to divide, it replicates its DNA in the part of interphase called the **S-phase** (S = synthesis). It is not known what causes transformation of a cell from the G_1 to the S phase.

Once there has been replication of DNA, the chromatin condenses into short, thick rodlike structures. It is in this form that chromosomes are more familiar to us as they can be seen with an ordinary light microscope.

Centrosomes are only found in cells that are capable of dividing. During cell division, centrioles position themselves on opposite sides of the nucleus. The centrioles then become involved in the producing of, and are attached to, spindle fibers. During cell division, the centrioles and spindle fibers pull the duplicated chromosomes to opposite poles of the cell. Any cell that lacks centrioles, such as mature nerve and muscle cells, cannot divide. It is during mitosis that cells are the most radiosensitive. The most radioresistant phase of the cell cycle is in late S-phase.

After the S-phase of the cell cycle, each chromosome includes two strands termed chromatids. The chromatids are connected together by a centromere. Within a chromosome the two chromatids bear identical DNA base sequences as each is made by DNA replication. Thus, each chromatid contains an entire double helix DNA molecule that is a duplicate of the single DNA molecule that existed before replication. Upon completion of cell division, each chromatid becomes a separate chromosome.

Following G_2, the gap or growth phase following the replication of DNA and prior to mitosis, the cell then enters into the four stages of cell division or mitosis (the M phase of the cell cycle). The stages of mitosis are **prophase, metaphase, anaphase,** and **telophase**.

Prophase   Chromosomes include two chromatids connected by a centromere. The centrioles migrate toward opposite poles of the cell, producing spindle fibers that extend across the cell's equator. The nuclear membrane begins to disappear, and the nucleolus is no longer visible.

Metaphase   The paired chromosomes are lined up at the equator of the cell. Spindle fibers from each centriole attach to the centromeres of the chromosomes. The nuclear membrane has entirely disappeared, and the centromeres now divide.

Anaphse   The centromeres divide, and the sister chromatids detach as they are pulled to an opposite pole. Each chromatid is regarded as a separate chromosome, as there are two complete and distinct sets.

Telophase   The sets of chromosomes become much longer, thinner, and indistinct as they reach the poles of the cell. The DNA unravels to form chromatin. There is formation of new nuclear membranes. The nucleolus reappears. Cytokinesis (cell division) is almost complete.

Once the cytoplasm divides, a new cell membrane is constructed, and two new daughter cells are formed. Figure 2-6 illustrates the process of mitosis.

Meiosis

In the formation of germ cells, a unique type of cell division transpires in the gonads (ovaries and testes) of sexually mature people. This type of cell division is termed meiosis. In the female, the specific meiotic process is labeled oogenesis. In the male, it is called spermatogenesis. Because ova and sperm have one-half the number of chromosomes, n (23), as the parent cell, 2n (46), meiosis is also referred to as reduction division. If a zygote is to include the diploid number (2n), it is essential that there is a reduction in

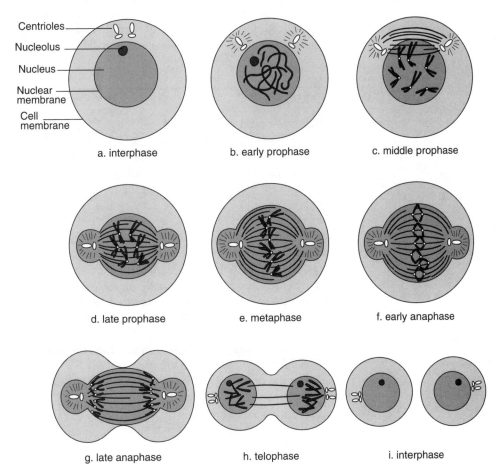

FIGURE 2–6
Mitosis

the chromosome number of germ cells. If there was not a reduction from 2n to n, this would mean the zygote would acquire two times the required number of chromosomes.

During meiosis, the cell divides twice in succession, but chromosomes are duplicated only once. In both germ and somatic cells, DNA synthesis takes place during interphase, with the result being a **duplication** of each chromosome constructing two chromatids. Thus, at the beginning of meiosis, a germ cell contains twice the amount of genetic material.

The names of the stages for meiosis and mitosis are the same. The movements of the germ cell chromosomes during meiosis are comparable to the way somatic cell chromosomes move during mitosis. At the completion of telophase, the original parent germ cell has created two daughter cells which contain the diploid or 2n (46) number of chromosomes. It is at this moment that the resemblances between meiosis and mitosis end.

The daughter cells now go through a second division of cellular material without replication of the DNA or duplication of the chromosomes. The result of these two successive divisions of meiosis is four gametes each of which contains the haploid number (23) of chromosomes. Figure 2–7 illustrates the process of meiosis.

KEY CONCEPTS

- A cell is composed of a cell membrane, cytoplasm, organelles, and a nucleus. Each has a distinct function. The cell membrane separates the interior of the cell from the exterior of the cell and surrounding cells. The cytoplasm is the site of chemical reactions within the cell. The organelles aid in the functioning of the cell. The nucleus is the brain of metabolic activity and cell division.
- There are four types of organic compounds: proteins, carbohydrates, lipids, and nucleic acids. Proteins assist in cellular growth and repair, carbohydrates provide energy to the cell, lipids provide energy storage, insulation and lubrication, and nucleic acids comprise the DNA and RNA of the cell.
- Potassium and sodium are inorganic molecules vital to cell life. These substances serve to maintain osmotic pressure within the cell.
- Mitosis is the process of cell division in which the nucleus and the cytoplasm divide to form two identical cells.
- Meiosis is the process of cell division for the purpose of reproduction.

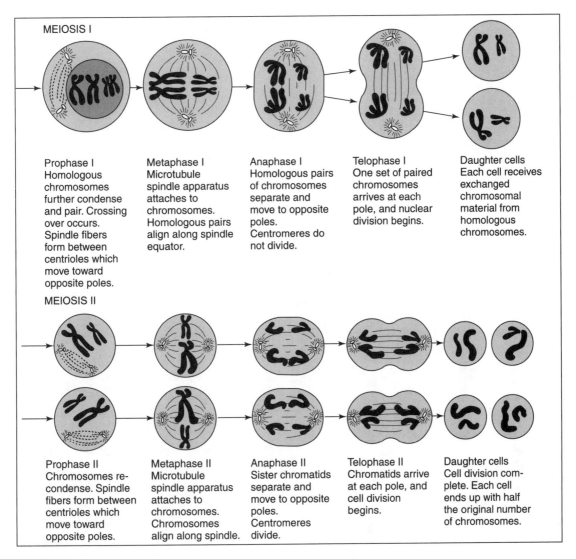

MEIOSIS I

Prophase I
Homologous chromosomes further condense and pair. Crossing over occurs. Spindle fibers form between centrioles which move toward opposite poles.

Metaphase I
Microtubule spindle apparatus attaches to chromosomes. Homologous pairs align along spindle equator.

Anaphase I
Homologous pairs of chromosomes separate and move to opposite poles. Centromeres do not divide.

Telophase I
One set of paired chromosomes arrives at each pole, and nuclear division begins.

Daughter cells
Each cell receives exchanged chromosomal material from homologous chromosomes.

MEIOSIS II

Prophase II
Chromosomes re-condense. Spindle fibers form between centrioles which move toward opposite poles.

Metaphase II
Microtubule spindle apparatus attaches to chromosomes. Chromosomes align along spindle.

Anaphase II
Sister chromatids separate and move to opposite poles. Centromeres divide.

Telophase II
Chromatids arrive at each pole, and cell division begins.

Daughter cells
Cell division complete. Each cell ends up with half the original number of chromosomes.

FIGURE 2–7
Meiosis

Cellular Effects of Radiation

KEY TERMS

Deletion

Dicentric

Division delay

Dose-response relationship (curve)

Effectiveness

Free radical

HeLa

Interphase death

Linear dose-response curve

Linear quadratic dose-response curve

Linear energy transfer (LET)

Mutation

Nonthreshold

Oxygen effect

Point mutation

Polyribosomes

Radiolysis

Radiosensitivity

Relative biologic effectiveness (RBE)

Ring

Sigmoid

System

Threshold

Translocation

OBJECTIVES

Upon completion of this chapter, the reader should be able to:

- Examine the physical and biologic factors affecting cell radiosensitivity
- Inspect the direct and indirect effects of radiation
- Evaluate the radiolysis of water
- Explain the irradiation of macromolecules
- Analyze the types of dose-response relationships
- Discuss the target theory
- Explain cell survival curves

RADIOSENSITIVITY OF CELLS

When radiation damage appears at the whole body level, this is a result of damage to organ **system**s, which are a consequence of radiation damage to cells of that particular system.

Tissue system cells are distinguished by their rate of cell division (proliferation), and their stage of development. *Immature cells are also known as undifferentiated, precursor, or stem cells.* As stated previously in the Law of Bergonie and Tribondeau, immature cells are significantly more radiosensitive than are mature cells.

Cells which are considered highly radiosensitive include: lymphocytes, spermatogonia, erythroblasts, and intestinal crypt cells.

Cells which have an intermediate radiosensitivity include: endothelial cells, osteoblasts, spermatids, and fibroblasts.

Cells which have low radiosensitivity include: muscle and nerve cells, and chondrocytes.

Cell radiosensitivity depends upon what part of the cell cycle the cell is in. Mitosis, and the passage from late G_1 into early S-phase, are judged the most radiosensitive phases of the cell cycle. Mid- to late S-phase is considered to be the most radioresistant cell cycle phase.

Numerous experiments have determined that the nucleus of a cell is considerably more radiosensitive than is the cytoplasm of the cell. DNA is the most radiosensitive part of the cell. RNA radiosensitivity is intermediate between that of DNA and protein. Chromosome produced radiation damage can be analyzed during the metaphase portion of the cell cycle.

Physical and Biologic Factors

When a cell is irradiated, three events may occur. These include the slowing down of cell mitosis, **interphase death**, and cell death.

It has been proven in experiments that low doses of radiation delay cell mitosis in humans. It is not known specifically what is the cause for this slow-down, known as division delay.

Interphase death, which is cell death before entering mitosis, is dependent on which cell is irradiated. Highly mitotic cells demonstrate interphase death at doses lower than cells that are not highly mitotic. It is theorized that when there is a change in the cell membrane, electrolytes become imbalanced. The consequence for cells that do not divide repetitively, or that divide numerous times resulting in dead cells being produced, is failure of cell reproduction.

When noting biologic changes that occur in cells caused by irradiating them, the following should be emphasized:

- Radiation interaction with cells has to do with chance and probability. The radiation may or may not interact; if it does interact, there may or may not be cell damage.
- The first deposit of radiation is given very rapidly, approximately within 10-17 seconds.
- The interaction of radiation within the cell is random.

- It cannot be determined if visible changes to cells, tissues, and organs is caused by radiation, or other sources.
- Radiation doses to cells cause biologic changes only following a period of time which is dose dependent, and may vary from minutes to years.

The factors affecting cell response include linear energy transfer (LET), relative biologic effectiveness (RBE), and oxygen enhancement ratio (OER).

Linear Energy Transfer   **Linear energy transfer (LET)** describes a measure of the rate at which energy is deposited as a charged particle travels through matter. LET is described in terms of keV/micrometer. LET is a function of the physical characteristics of radiation, that is, mass and charge. As electromagnetic radiation (x- and gamma-rays) produce few and sparse interactions because of their fast moving electrons (which have negligible mass and a -1 charge), they are regarded as low LET radiation. These lose or deposit their energy at a much lower rate when passing through tissue.

Compared with electromagnetic radiation, particulate radiations (e.g., alpha particles and neutrons), which are highly ionizing and have substantial mass and/or charge, are more likely to interact with tissue. These radiations lose their energy quickly, and produce numerous ionizations within a very short distance. Alpha and neutron radiation are thus considered high LET radiations.

The higher the LET of radiation, the greater the chance for a biologic interaction. Diagnostic x-rays, which have an LET of approximately 3 keV/μm, are considered to be low when compared with all radiations.

Table 3–1 lists average LET values for different types of radiation.

TABLE 3-1

TYPES OF RADIATION WITH CORRESPONDING LET VALUES	
RADIATION TYPE	**LET (keV/μm)**
Cobalt-60	0.25
1 MeV electrons	0.3
Diagnostic x-rays	3.0
10 MeV protons	4.0
2.5 MeV neutrons	20.0
5 MeV alpha particle	100.0
Heavy nuclei	1000.0

Relative Biologic Effectiveness   The relative effect of LET is quantitatively described by the **relative biologic effectiveness (RBE)**. RBE is a comparison of a dose of test radiation to a dose of 250 keV x-ray which produces the same biologic response. RBE is expressed as follows:

$$RBE = \frac{\text{dose in rads from 250 keV x-ray necessary to produce a given effect}}{\text{dose in rads of test radiation necessary to produce the same effect}}$$

The constant is the biologic response, not the radiation dose. The RBE measures the biologic effectiveness of radiations having different LET's.

EXAMPLE

When rats are irradiated with 250 kEv x-rays, 300 rad are required to cause death. If these rats are irradiated with heavy nuclei, only 100 rad are necessary. Calculate the RBE for the heavy nuclei.

$$RBE = \frac{300 \text{ rad}}{100 \text{ rad}} = 3$$

Factors which influence RBE include radiation type, cell or tissue type, physiologic condition, biologic result being examined, and the radiation dose rate.

In comparing LET and RBE, as LET increases, RBE increases also (see Figure 3–1). Accordingly, low LET radiations have a low RBE, and

FIGURE 3–1
RBE vs. LET

high LET radiations have a high RBE. Diagnostic x-rays are considered to have an RBE of approximately 1.

Oxygen Enhancement Ratio   The response of biologic tissue to radiation is greater when irradiated in the oxygenated, or aerobic state than when irradiated in anoxic or hypoxic conditions. This is known as the **oxygen effect**. The oxygen effect is described numerically by the oxygen enhancement ratio (OER). OER is defined as the dose of radiation that produces a given biologic response under anoxic conditions divided by the dose of radiation that produces the same biologic response under aerobic conditions. It is theorized that oxygen is needed in order for free radicals to form during ionization of water. Without the free radicals, hydrogen peroxide is not formed, and thus cell damage is reduced.

$$OER = \frac{\text{dose that produces a given biologic response under anoxic conditions}}{\text{dose that produces the same biologic response under aerobic conditions}}$$

OER is dependent on LET. The OER is most pronounced for low LET radiation, and is less effective with high LET radiation. For mammal cells, OER is between 2 and 3. The OER for high LET radiations is between 1.2 and 1.7.

Because of the physical differences between high and low LET radiation, the quantity of damage done by high LET radiation would be beyond repair. Thus, having oxygen present would not intensify the response to radiation to the same magnitude, as would be the case with low LET radiation (see Figure 3–2).

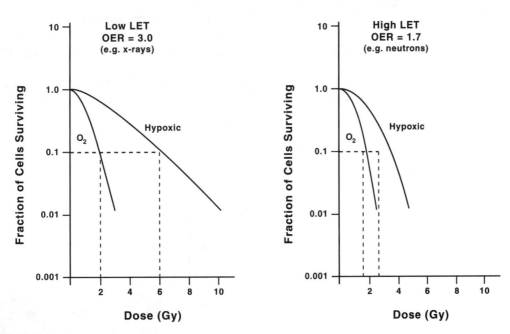

FIGURE 3–2
Oxygen effect on LET

EXAMPLE

Rat tumors are irradiated using hypoxic conditions. The tumor control dose is 5,000 rad. Irradiating the tumors under aerobic conditions requires a control dose of 1,000 rad. What is the OER for this system?

$$OER = \frac{5,000}{1,000} = 5$$

Age   Age influences radiosensitivity. We are most radiosensitive before birth. Radiosensitivity declines until maturity, the time when we are most radioresistant. With old age humans again tend to become more radiosensitive (see Figure 3–3). These concepts are consistent with the law of Bergonie and Tribondeau.

Gender   Experiments have shown that females can tolerate approximately 5–10% more radiation than males. Accordingly, men are more radiosensitive than women.

Direct and Indirect Effects of Radiation

When radiation interactions occur in a cell, these ionizations and excitations develop either in macromolecules, (e.g., DNA) or in their suspension medium (e.g., water). Depending on the location of the interaction, it is termed either direct or indirect.

Direct interaction is said to take place when an original ionizing incident happens on that macromolecule (e.g., DNA, RNA, protein or enzyme). If a macromolecule becomes ionized, it is considered abnormal and thus damaged.

Indirect interaction occurs if the initial ionizing incident takes place on a distant noncritical molecule, which then transfers the ionization of energy to another molecule.

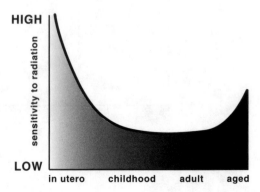

FIGURE 3–3
Age and radiosensitivity

INTERACTIONS WITH RADIATION

Although it is impossible to determine whether ionizations of molecules occur through direct versus indirect effects, as the human body is approximately 80% water, it is theorized that most radiation actions with humans are indirect. The response to cell irradiation is also determined by the dose in rads.

Radiolysis of Water

With the human body being approximately 80% water, it follows that the irradiation of water is involved in the majority of interactions involving radiation. Although DNA is the most critical target of radiation, it is the irradiation of water, which causes indirect effects, that is the principal cause of effects from radiation. If water is irradiated, the water is ionized, and separates into other molecular products. This is called the **radiolysis** of water.

When an atom of water is irradiated, this ionizes the water, and produces a **free radical** (Figure 3–4). A free radical is an uncharged molecule that contains a single unpaired electron in its outermost or valence shell, which makes it chemically unstable and highly reactive.

Even though free radicals have an estimated life of less than 1 millisecond, they are able to diffuse through the cell and interact at a distant site. They have excess energy which can be moved to other molecules and interfere with bonds at sites distant from the original ionizing incident. Reactions of water include:

$H_2O + radiation = HOH^+ + e^-$
$H_2O + e^- = HOH^-$
$HOH^+ = H^+ + OH^*$
$HOH^- = OH^- + H^*$
$OH^* + OH^* = H_2O_2$

The end result of the radiolysis of water is the development of an ion pair, H^+ and OH^-, and two free radicals, H^* and OH^*. The ions can recombine and form a normal water molecule, or they can react chemically and damage cell macromolecules.

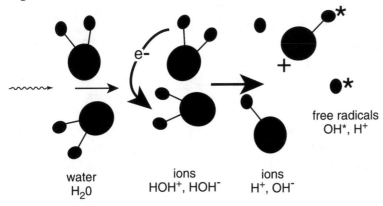

| water
H_2O | ions
HOH^+, HOH^- | ions
H^+, OH^- | free radicals
OH^*, H^+ |

FIGURE 3–4
Free radical formation

The OH*, which is the hydroxyl free radical, along with hydrogen peroxide (H_2O_2) is estimated to cause approximately two-thirds of all radiation damage following the radiolysis of water.

Ionization occurs when an atom has an extra electron, or has had an electron removed. If an ion has more electrons than it does protons, it is designated with a negative sign. If an ion has more protons than electrons, it is designated with a positive sign.

Irradiation of Macromolecules

The occurrence of molecular derangements or lesions may be classified as either effects on macromolecules or effects on water. Irradiating macromolecules gives very different results when compared to the irradiating of water [Figure 3–5]. If macromolecules are exposed to ionizing radiation in vitro (outside the body or cell), a significant dose of radiation is needed to produce a measurable effect. Irradiating macromolecules in vivo (inside the living cell) shows that when cells are in their natural conditions, they are much more radiosensitive.

The three primary effects of irradiating macromolecules in vitro include main-chain scission, cross-linking, and point lesions.

Main-chain Scission   Main-chain scission occurs when the thread or backbone of the long-chain molecule is broken. This results in the long-chain molecule being reduced to numerous smaller molecules, which can still be macromolecular in nature. Not only is the size of the macromolecule reduced, but its viscosity (thickness) is also reduced.

FIGURE 3–5
Macromolecule
mutations

A.   B.   C.

Cross-linking Certain macromolecules have spurlike extensions off the main chain. Others develop these spurs after being irradiated. After being irradiated, these spurs can act as if they had sticky material on their ends. This stickiness causes the macromolecule to connect to another macromolecule, or to another section of the same molecule. This is termed cross-linking. Viscosity is increased by radiation-produced molecular cross-linking.

Point Lesions Irradiating macromolecules may result in disturbance of single chemical bonds, which create molecular lesions or point lesions. Point lesions may cause slight molecular changes, which in turn cause the cell to function incorrectly.

At low doses of radiation, point lesions are regarded to be the cellular radiation damage that is responsible for the late radiation effects, which are observed at the whole-body level.

Irradiating macromolecules may result in either death of the cell or late effects. Throughout the cell cycle proteins are constantly being created, and occur in greater numbers than the nucleic acids. Abundant copies of unique protein molecules always exist in the cell. These factors allow proteins to be more radioresistant than the nucleic acids. Also, numerous copies of m-RNA and t-RNA exist in the cell, although they are not as plentiful as the protein molecules. Conversely, DNA molecules, having their distinctive base arrangements, are not so numerous. Because of this, DNA is considered the most radiosensitive macromolecule. RNA **radiosensitivity** is midway between that of DNA and protein macromolecules.

There can be visible chromosome abnormalities or cytogenetic damage if the radiation damage to the DNA is intense enough. DNA can be injured without producing visible chromosomal aberrations. Even though this damage is reversible, it can lead to death of the cell, and ultimately destroy tissues or organs.

Metabolic activity can also be affected by DNA damage. The primary characteristic of radiation-induced malignancies is the uncontrolled reproduction of cells. If germ cells receive DNA damage, the response may be detected in future offspring.

Figure 3–6 A–D illustrates DNA aberrations that are all reversible types of damage. They may involve the sequence of bases being changed, thus changing the triplet code of codons. This is considered a genetic mutation at the molecular level.

Damage type shown in Figure 3–6E also involves the change of or loss of a base. This type of damage also destroys the triplet code, and may not be reversible; this is considered a genetic mutation.

These molecular genetic **mutations** are termed **point mutations**, and are common with low LET radiations. Point mutations may be either of minor or major significance to the cell. A very major effect of these point mutations would be the genetic code being incorrectly transferred to daughter cells.

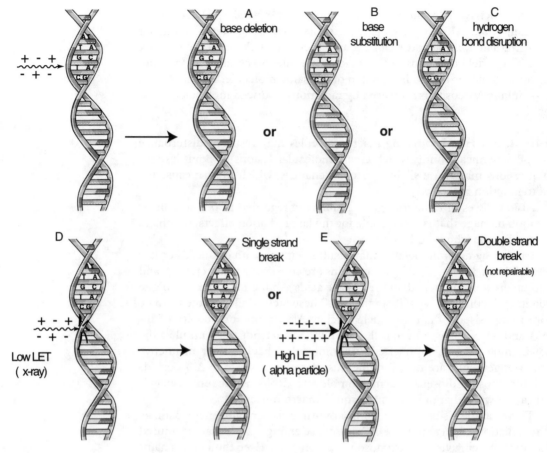

FIGURE 3–6
DNA aberrations

Single-hit Chromosome Aberrations

When chromosomes are irradiated, the interaction can be either direct or indirect. The result of either interaction is called a hit. Chromosome hits cause a visible chromosome change (Figure 3–7). Such a hit would mean numerous molecular bonds had been interfered with, and that several chains of DNA had been severed. Chromosome hits represent critical DNA damage.

Figure 3–8 demonstrates the single-hit effects caused by radiation during the G_1 portion of the cell cycle.

If there is breakage of a chromatid, this is termed chromatid **deletion**. During the S-phase of the cell cycle, the deletion and the remaining chromosome are replicated. The chromosome abnormality which is seen during metaphase is a normal appearing chromosome with material missing from the ends of two sister chromatids and two acentric fragments. These type of fragments are called isochromatids.

	Breakage	Recombination	Replication	Anaphasic Separation
A. One break in one chromosome		NONE		
B. Two breaks in one chromosome Rings				or
C. One break in two chromosomes Translocation				
D. One break in two chromosomes Dicentrics				

FIGURE 3–7
Chromosome aberrations (Reprinted with permission from Bushong. [1997]. *Radiologic science for technologists* [6th ed.]. St. Louis: Mosby.)

Chromosome aberrations from single-hit events can also happen during the G_2 phase of the cell cycle (see Figure 3–9).

There is a low probability that ionizing radiation will pass through sister chromatids to produce isochromatids. Instead, the radiation normally causes a chromatid deletion in just one arm of the chromosome. This results in a chromosome arm which is missing a chromatid fragment and consequently is missing genetic material.

G_1 irradiation in G_1 causes chromatid break   that is replicated in S and passed through G_2 to be seen at M

FIGURE 3–8
Single hit affects G_1 (Reprinted with permission from Bushong. [1997]. *Radiologic science for technologists* [6th ed.]. St. Louis: Mosby.)

FIGURE 3–9

Single hit affects G_2 (Reprinted with permission from Bushong. [1997]. *Radiologic science for technologists* [6th ed.]. St. Louis: Mosby.)

Multi-hit Chromosome Aberrations

It is theorized that human chromosomes have more than a single target. Thus, it is feasible for a single chromosome to receive more than one hit (Figure 3–10). These multi-hit aberrations are not unusual.

During the G_1 phase of the cell cycle, if two hits occur on one chromosome, **ring** chromosomes are produced. When neighboring chromosomes each suffer one hit and then recombine, this produces **dicentric (a chromosome with two centers or two centromeres)** fragments. The quality of the stickiness present at the severed chromosome is the determining factor for the joining of the chromatids (see Figure 3–10).

During the G_2 phase of the cell cycle, similar chromosomal abnormalities can occur. These types of aberrations are rare, as they require that the same chromosome is hit two or more times, or that neighboring chromosomes are hit and join together.

Multi-hit chromosomal aberrations are representative of major cell damage. During mitosis, either the acentric fragments will be lost, or they

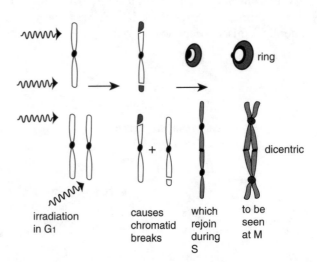

FIGURE 3–10

Multi–hit chromosome aberrations. (Reprinted with permission from Bushong. [1997]. *Radiologic science for technologists* [6th ed.]. St. Louis: Mosby.)

will be attracted to just one of the two daughter cells, as they are not connected to a spindle fiber. This results in one or both daughter cells missing significant genetic information.

Reciprocal Translocations

Reciprocal **translocation**s are multi-hit chromosomal aberrations. If chromosomes experience this type of alteration, they do not lose any genetic material, but instead the genes become rearranged. This results in all genetic codes being available, but sequenced incorrectly (see Figure 3–11).

At the doses received in diagnostic radiology, only single-hit types of chromosomal aberrations are seen. If the radiation dose is not known, the approximate chromosomal aberration frequency will be: two single-hit aberrations/rad/1000 cells, and one multi-hit aberration/10 rad/1000 cells.

DOSE–RESPONSE RELATIONSHIPS

Dose-response relationships, also referred to as dose-response curves, are a graphical relationship between observed effects (response) from radiation and dose of radiation received (Figure 3–12).

Dose-response curves differ in two ways:

1. They are either linear or nonlinear
2. They are either threshold or nonthreshold

Linear means that an observed response is directly proportional to the dose.

EXAMPLE

Doubling the dose of radiation would double the response.

Nonlinear means that an observed response is not directly proportional to the dose.

EXAMPLE

Doubling the dose of radiation does not double the response.

FIGURE 3–11
Reciprocal translocations. (Reprinted with permission from Bushong. [1997]. *Radiologic science for technologists* [6th ed.]. St. Louis: Mosby.)

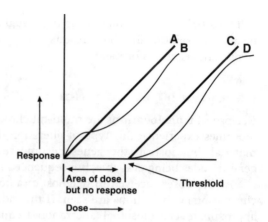

FIGURE 3–12
Dose–response relationships

Threshold assumes that there is a radiation level reached below which there would be no effects observed. **Nonthreshold** assumes that any radiation dose produces an effect.

Diagnostic radiology is primarily concerned with linear, nonthreshold dose-response relationships.

Linear–Dose-Response Relationships

Since dose-response relationships A and B intercept the dose (x) axis at either zero or on the y-axis, they are considered linear, nonthreshold (see Figure 3–12).

All linear dose-response relationships exhibit an effect regardless of the dose. This is demonstrated by relationship A. Even at zero dose, A exhibits a measurable response, R_A. This R_A is termed the ambient or natural response. Dose-response relationships C and D intercept the dose (x) axis at a dose value greater than zero. Thus, C and D are considered linear, threshold. At doses below the respective C and D values, no response would be anticipated.

Leukemia, breast cancer, and other genetic damage are believed to follow the linear dose-response relationship.

Linear Quadratic Dose–Response Curves

In 1980 the Committee on the Biological Effects of Ionizing Radiation (BEIR Committee) concluded that the effects of low doses of low LET radiation follow a **linear, quadratic dose–response** relationship (Figure 3–13). At low doses, the curve is linear. At higher doses, the curve becomes curvilinear. The curve is nonthreshold.

The portion of the curve where increases in dose show no or little increase in effect is named the toe. The shoulder is considered the area of the curve in which a leveling off occurs, again demonstrating no or little increase in effect.

This model underestimates the low dose effect of radiation, as the linear part of the curve is somewhat leveled off or flattened.

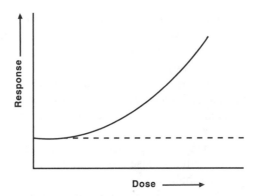

FIGURE 3–13
Linear quadratic dose-response
curve

In 1990, with 10 additional years of human data, the BEIR committee revised its radiation risk estimates and adopted the linear, nonthreshold dose-response relationship as most relevant.

Current radiation protection guidelines are established using the linear nonthreshold dose-response relationship model.

Nonlinear Dose–Response Relationships   The sigmoid dose-response curve is applied predominately to the high dose effects observed in radiotherapy (Figure 3–14). Sigmoid means s-shaped. There is normally a threshold below which no observable effects occur.

With a sigmoid dose-response curve, there is a nonlinear relationship between dose and effect, meaning that the effect is not directly proportional to the dose.

TARGET THEORY

As cells contain a profusion of molecules, radiation damage to these molecules is not likely to result in significant cell injury because additional molecules are present to assist in cell survival. However, there are molecules that are not in abundance which are considered necessary for cell survival. Irradiating these could have serious consequences, because there may not be others available to maintain cell survival.

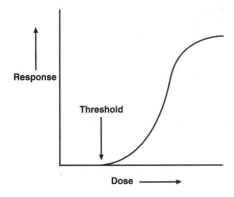

FIGURE 3–14
Sigmoid dose-response curve

This idea of a sensitive critical molecule is the foundation for the target theory. According to the target theory, there will be cell death only if the cell's target molecule is inactivated. It is theorized that DNA is the critical molecular target.

The target is regarded to be the area of the cell that contains the target molecule. Because radiation interaction with cells is random, target interactions also occur randomly. The radiation shows no favoritism toward the target molecule.

When a target is irradiated, this is considered a hit. Both direct and indirect effects cause hits (Figure 3–15). Direct vversus indirect hits are not distinguishable.

With low LET radiation in an anoxic condition, chances for a hit on the target molecule are low because of the large distances between ionizing events.

In an aerobic state with low LET radiation, the indirect effect is intensified, as more free radicals are formed, and the volume of action surrounding each interaction is enlarged. This increases the likelihood of a hit.

Using high LET radiation, ionization distances are so close together that there is a high probability that a direct hit will take place, probably even higher than for the low LET, indirect effect.

FIGURE 3–15

Target theory (Reproduced with permission from Bushberg, J.T., Seibert, J.A., Leidholt, E.M., and Boone, J. M., [2001]. *The essential physics of medical imaging* [2nd ed.]. Philadelphia: Lippincott, Williams and Wilkins.

Adding oxygen to high LET radiation will probably not result in additional hits, as the high LET has already produced the maximum number of hits possible.

CELL SURVIVAL CURVES

Cellular sensitivity studies began in the middle 1950s with Puck and Marcus. They performed in vitro studies using **HeLa** cells. Their initial study was on failure of reproduction in which they exposed HeLa cells to differing radiation doses and then totaled the number of colonies formed.

This information may be illustrated graphically by plotting the radiation doses on a linear scale on the x-axis, and plotting the fraction of surviving cells on a logarithmic scale on the y-axis. This graphical representation of the relationship between dose and surviving cells is a cell survival curve.

It was stated previously that radiation interaction is random in nature. Therefore, we must determine how many hits are necessary to cause cell death. This may be demonstrated using a cell survival curve.

In simple cells such as bacteria, if there are additional hits to the same cell, these hits do not matter. In complex cells such as human cells, it is theorized that in order to cause cell death, more than one hit is required.

The graphs of simple versus complex cells are very different (see Figure 3–16).

Graph A represents a survival curve for simple cells, represented by a straight line.

Graph B represents a survival curve for complex cells, represented by a line which displays a shouldered area where effects are not apparent until some targets have received enough multiple hits to be killed. The target theory can be used to explain this shoulder section of the curve.

If there are n number of cell targets, for example, n = 5, all have to be hit for a cell to be killed. Therefore, the cell must receive 5 sublethal hits to cause cell death, otherwise the cell will be able to repair itself. The shoulder region of the curve is the area where hits = n - 1 (e.g., 5 - 1), or 4 hits for each cell.

The shoulder of the cell survival curve shows that some damage must accrue before there can be cell death. The accumulated damage is called sublethal damage. The wider the shoulder, the more sublethal damage the cell can endure.

KEY CONCEPTS

- Radiation causes a slowdown in cell mitosis, interphase death of cells prior to mitosis, and cell death. Cells are most radiosensitive when they are young and when they are undergoing mitosis.
- Direct radiation occurs when the ionizing incident occurs on a particular macromolecule. Indirect radiation occurs when the ionizing

FIGURE 3–16
Simple versus complex cell survival curves

incident occurs on a macromolecule distant from the macromolecule affected by the radiation.

- The majority of interactions involving radiation in the human are the result of irradiation of water in the cells that becomes ionized and separates into other molecular products.

- Radiation of macromolecules has three effects: (1) main-chain scission in which the macromolecule is reduced in size and thickness, (2) cross-linking in which the spurs on the macromolecule adhere to other macromolecules enlarging and thickening the original macromolecule, and (3) point lesions in which slight molecular changes occur that cause the cell to function incorrectly.

- In linear dose-response relationships effects of radiation are exhibited regardless of the dose. In linear quadratic dose-response relationships a leveling off effect is observed as doses are increased. Nonlinear dose-response relationships show effects that are not directly proportional to the dose.

- The target theory suggests that there are sensitive critical molecules that are essential to cell survival and that radiation to these cells will result in cell death.

- The cell survival curve identifies the doses that result in inability of the cell to reproduce thus leading to cell death.

SECTION REVIEW

1. The process of cell division of somatic cells is known as:
   a. mitosis
   b. synthesis
   c. meiosis
   d. reduction division

2. How does oxygen retention affect cell radiosensitivity?
   a. increases radiosensitivity
   b. decreases radiosensitivity
   c. destroys radiosensitivity
   d. does not affect radiosensitivity

3. What is the name of the molecule that has one or more unpaired electrons and is usually chemically reactive?
   a. centromere
   b. polypeptide
   c. free radical
   d. ion

4. Which of the following measures the rate of energy lost along the track of an ionizing particle?
   a. relative biologic effectiveness (RBE)
   b. linear energy transfer (LET)
   c. oxygen enhancement ratio (OER)
   d. cell survival curve

5. Which of the following would be considered most radiosensitive?
   a. a fetus
   b. a pediatric patient
   c. a teenage patient
   d. an adult patient

CASE STUDY

A 22-year-old female is scheduled for a barium enema study. As you are taking her patient history, she informs you there is a possibility she might be pregnant. Discuss how the law of Bergonie and Tribondeau could determine the radiologist's decision on whether to perform the exam on your patient.

Biological Effects of Radiation Exposure

It is crucial that radiographers study the effects of ionizing radiation. Radiographers must comprehend the potential risks of ionizing radiation by acquiring a thorough understanding of radiation biology. This section discusses the clinical applications of radiation biology.

Effects of radiation exposure that occur within minutes, hours, days and weeks are termed early effects. In contrast, late effects of radiation exposure occur months and even years later.

The manner in which an organism responds to total body radiation is determined by the combined response of all the body systems. Since body systems differ in both radiosensitivity and response, total body response is a function of the specific system which is most influenced by the exposure to radiation.

Effects of Initial Exposure to Radiation

KEY TERMS

Aberration

Acentric

Alopecia

Anemia

Anomaly

Atrophy

Crypts of Lieberkuhn

Cytopenia

Dermis

Desquamation

Dicentric

Edema

Epidermis

Erythroblasts

Follicles

Granulocytes

Hemopoietic

Inflammation

Karyotype

Latent

LD50/30

LD50/60

Lesion

Manifest

Maturation depletion

Megakaryocytes

Meningitis

Myelocytes

Necrosis

Oogonia

Prodromal

Radiation cataractogenesis

Radioresistant

Sebaceous

SED50

Skin erythema dose (SED)

Somatic

Spermatogonia

Stem cell

Stroma

Subcutaneous

Syndrome

Threshold dose

Vasculitis

OBJECTIVES

Upon completion of this chapter, the reader should be able to:

- Discuss the hematologic, gastrointestinal, and central nervous system syndromes
- Describe local tissue damage to the skin, eyes and gonads
- Explain hematologic and cytogenetic effects

ACUTE RADIATION SYNDROMES

After an organism is exposed to acute whole body radiation, it exhibits certain signs, symptoms and clinical findings. The term syndrome is used to show the relationship of the signs and symptoms to a specific type of trauma or disease process. The term total body radiation syndrome is used as the response of an organism to whole body radiation results in specific findings. Even though the syndrome is caused by damage to one specific system, presentation of unique signs and symptoms are caused by damage to more than one body system.

In order for the total body radiation syndrome to be applicable, radiation exposure must happen under the following conditions: 1) an organ must have been exposed acutely, that is, in a matter of seconds or minutes; 2) there must be exposure of the total body area; 3) external penetrating sources, for example, x-rays, gamma-rays, and neutrons, produce the radiation syndromes. Internally deposited radioactive materials do not result in manifestation of the full syndrome.

The main consequence of an acute radiation exposure is shortening of the life span of the organism. This life span shortening is dose dependent. Because the life span of an organism is dramatically decreased after a moderate to high dose of total body radiation (many hundreds or thousands of rads), whole body exposures in this dose range are regarded as instantly fatal.

Organism survival times are expressed as the average survival time. There are variations in survival times between different species and between animals within the same species. Expressing survival time as the average takes these variations into account.

Because of the variations in survival time of a group of animals exposed to the same whole body dose, the relationship of survival of a whole population of the same species exposed to the same dose is expressed as that dose which will kill a certain percentage of the population within a given period of time. For example the lethal dose required to kill 50% of a population in 30 days is expressed as the **LD50/30**. As humans often survive beyond this 30-day period, the **LD50/60**, or the lethal dose required to kill 50% of a population in 60 days, may be more useful. The LD50/60 is approximately 250–300 rads. The LD50/30 and acute radiation syndromes assume no medical intervention. Table 4–1 lists the LD50/30 doses in rads for various species:

A curve can be made which relates dose to survival time for all mammals exposed to whole body radiation (Figure 4–1). As dose goes up, the survival time and number of survivors decreases.

In the dose range of 200 R, death occurs in a small percentage of animals, with the survival time being dose dependent. Animals exposed in this range survive a few weeks. Between 1,000 and 10,000 R, average survival time does not appear to be dose dependent. In this range, all animals irradiated survive about the same time, approximately 3–4 days, but fewer survive at these doses than at the lower dose. At doses of 10,000 R and above, average survival time becomes dose dependent, with survival rate decreasing to hours or minutes.

TABLE 4–1

LD50/30 VALUES	
Species	**LD50/30 (rads)**
human	250–450
dog	300
monkey	400
chicken	600
frog	700
rabbit	800
rat	900
turtle	1,500
goldfish	2,000
newt	3,000

In referring to the three regions of the dose response curve, there are three different systems which can result in death to the animal. Other organs and systems have suffered damage, but the principal cause of death is destruction to one specific system. The three defined acute radiation syndromes are named corresponding to failure of that organ system which causes death. These doses are not likely to occur in diagnostic radiology.

In the 100 to 1,000 R range, death is mostly the result of damage to the **hemopoietic** (development of blood cells) system, especially to the bone

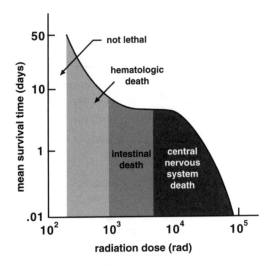

FIGURE 4–1

Mammalian dose survival curve

marrow. Thus, the acute radiation syndrome in this dose range is termed the hematologic, hematopoietic, or bone marrow syndrome.

In the second region of the dose response curve, at approximately 600 to 10,000 R, death is caused by damage to the gastrointestinal system, especially the small intestine. The syndrome within this dose range is known as the gastrointestinal (GI) syndrome.

The third region of the dose response curve, at doses greater than 10,000 R, death is caused by damage to the central nervous system. Thus, this third syndrome is called the central nervous system (CNS) syndrome.

It is important to note two specifics concerning the acute radiation syndrome dose response curve: 1) the dose range figures are obtained from studies of animal response after acute total body exposure, and are not specific for humans; 2) at the higher doses of each range, the syndromes overlap, for example, animals may die from a combination of damage in the bone marrow and GI syndromes. Figure 4–2 shows the interrelationships between the elements of the acute radiation syndrome.

FIGURE 4–2

Elements of acute radiation syndrome (Reproduced with permission from Bushberg, J. T., Seibert, J. A., Leidholt, E. M., and Boone, J. M. [2001]. *The essential physics of medical imaging.* [2nd ed.]. Philadelphia: Lippincott, Williams and Wilkins.

Response Stages

Animal responses to acute total body radiation doses are divided into four stages. The time length of each stage is dose dependent, that is, the lower the dose, the longer the duration in the stage. Each stage can last from weeks at low doses to minutes at high doses.

The first stage, termed the **prodromal** stage, consists of nausea, vomiting, and diarrhea (also referred to as the N-V-D syndrome). This stage, which can occur with a dose as low as 50 rads, lasts from a few minutes to a few days, being dose dependent (i.e., the higher the dose, the shorter the stage). Table 4–2 shows approximate doses in air that will cause various prodromal symptoms in 50% of those people irradiated.

The second stage is known as the **latent** stage. During this period, the animal appears to be symptom-free. In reality, changes are taking place that will either lead to recovery or death. The time length of this stage is also dose dependent, ranging from weeks as in doses below 500 R, to hours or less at doses greater than 10,000 R.

After the latent stage, the animal becomes noticeably ill and shows signs and symptoms of the specific syndrome reflecting the organ system which is damaged. This third stage is called the **manifest** illness stage, and lasts from minutes to weeks depending on the dose.

In the fourth stage, the animal either recovers or dies as a result of the damage sustained from the radiation exposure. Figure 4–3 summarizes the different phases of the acute radiation syndrome.

Even though the timing and manifestation of the signs and symptoms vary among various mammals, most mammals show similar signs and symptoms. The survival time after different doses differs greatly among species. In referring back to the LD50/30 values for different species, humans appear to be relatively radiosensitive.

TABLE 4–2

AIR DOSE CAUSING PRODROMAL SYMPTOMS	
Dose in Air	Symptoms
1.2 Gy (120 rads)	Anorexia
1.7 Gy (170 rads)	Nausea
2.1 Gy (210 rads)	Vomiting
2.4 Gy (240 rads)	Diarrhea

Pizzarello, D. J., & Witcofski, R. L. (1982) *Medical radiation biology* (2nd ed.) Philadelphia: Lea & Febiger.

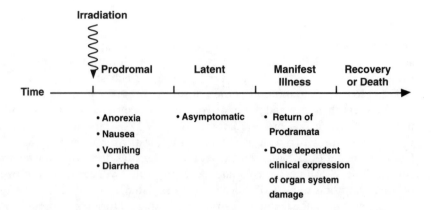

FIG 4–3
Acute radiation syndrome phases
(From Pizzarello, D. J., & Witcof-
ski, R. L. [1982]. *Medical radiation
biology* [2nd Ed.]. Philadelphia:
Lea & Febiger.)

Bone Marrow Syndrome

Bone marrow syndrome, also referred to as the hematologic or hematopoietic syndrome, occurs between 100 and 1,000 R, with death occurring
within 6–8 weeks in some individuals at a dose of 200 R. No one has survived a dose of 1,000 R. An exposure to this dose would cause death within
two weeks. The LD50/60 for humans is estimated to be about 450 R or
250–300 rads, and is in the dose range of this syndrome. Death is caused by
destruction of the bone marrow. The mechanism of death is caused by the
reduction of red blood cells (RBCs), white blood cells (WBCs), and
platelets. Death results from anemia and infection.

The prodromal stage of this syndrome occurs a few hours after exposure and involves nausea and vomiting. The latent stage extends from a few
days up to 3 weeks after exposure, during which time the number of circulating blood cells are not severely depressed. Even though the person looks
and feels well, in reality bone marrow stem cells are dying during the prodromal and latent stages. This results in fewer mature cells being produced
and lower numbers of cells in the circulating blood. Reduction in blood cell
count occurs during the manifest illness stage, which occurs at 3–5 weeks
postexposure. The signs and symptoms of the manifest illness stage include
depression of all blood cell counts (**cytopenia**), which causes **anemia** and
infections.

For people suffering with this syndrome, survival time is dose dependent. In the range of 100-300 R, the bone marrow repopulates enough to
sustain life in most individuals. A large percentage of these people will fully
recover during the 3rd week to 6 months postexposure. Doses from 400 to
600 R result in fewer survivors. No one has survived a dose of 1,000 R.

Assuming no medical intervention, death occurs in approximately 4–6
weeks in the 300 to 500 R range, but in 2 weeks in the 500 to 1,000 R dose
range. Destruction of the bone marrow causes infection and hemorrhage,
which ultimately leads to death at these doses. Normally the bone marrow is
filled with cells which supply the circulating blood with mature cells. After
exposures in this dose range, the number of bone marrow cells decreases

until the bone marrow is no longer able to produce the cells which are needed in the circulating blood to support life.

Gastrointestinal Syndrome

The gastrointestinal (GI) syndrome appears in all animals at doses between 1000 and 10,000 R. In humans, some symptoms appear at a **threshold dose** of 600 R, with the full syndrome manifest at 1,000 R. Survival time in this syndrome does not vary with dose. Death happens at the same time regardless of dose. Human death occurs within 3 to 10 days without medical support and within approximately 2 weeks with medical intervention.

Within hours after exposure the prodromal stage occurs. This stage involves nausea and vomiting, cramps, and diarrhea. The latent stage occurs through the fifth day. Following this stage there is a reoccurrence of nausea, vomiting and diarrhea along with a fever, which is the start of the manifest illness stage, which perseveres from the fifth through the tenth days.

The GI syndrome occurs because of damage to the GI tract and bone marrow. The GI tract lining, especially the small intestine, is damaged by doses in this range. Exposure to radiation causes the **crypts of Lieberkuhn** (the radiosensitive cells precursor to the population of villi cells) to be depleted. This causes the villi to lose cells, and becoming shortened, flattened and partly or completely denuded.

Because of the villi being flattened, there is decreased absorption of materials across the wall of the intestine. Dehydration occurs from fluids leaking into the GI tract lumen. Systemic infection results from bacteria that pass through the intestinal wall and enter the bloodstream.

During these changes to the GI tract, there is also a depletion of circulating white blood cells because of the bacteria entering the blood stream from the GI tract.

Even though the GI tract attempts regeneration after irradiation, the damage suffered by the bone marrow will likely still cause death. Death results from infection, dehydration and electrolyte imbalance caused by the damage sustained to the GI tract and bone marrow.

Central Nervous System Syndrome

The central nervous system (CNS) syndrome occurs at doses greater than 5,000 R in humans. Death is usually within hours, but may occur 2–3 days postexposure. Depending on the dose, the prodromal stage lasts from a few minutes to a few hours. The person suffers nervousness, confusion, nausea and vomiting, a loss of consciousness, and burning sensations of the skin. A latent period may last several hours. Manifest illness occurs 5–6 hours after exposure, resulting in diarrhea, convulsions, coma and death.

Death caused by the CNS syndrome is not fully understood. CNS damage may result from damage to the blood vessels that supply the system, thus causing **edema** (swelling) in the cranial vault, **vasculitis** (inflammation of blood vessels), and **meningitis** (inflammation of the spinal cord and brain membranes). It is thought that death is caused by increased pressure in the cranial vault as a result of elevated fluid content from the previously mentioned changes.

Even though the hematopoietic and GI syndromes are taking place, the person does not live long enough to exhibit these syndromes.

Table 4–3 summarizes the stages, dose range, major clinical symptoms, and effect of medical intervention on the acute radiation syndrome.

LOCAL TISSUE DAMAGE

All organs and body tissues can be affected by partial body irradiation. The result is death to some of the cells, which results in **atrophy** (shrinking) of the tissue or organ. This in turn may lead to that organ or tissue becoming nonfunctional, or to recovery. With high enough doses, any local tissue will react. Tissue response is dependent on its radiosensitivity, reproduction and maturation rates. The skin, gonads and extremities are examples of local tissues that can be affected.

Skin

Because of the early uses of radiation and radiation therapy, the skin is the tissue that we have a good deal of data about. During the early years of radiology, because of the low x-ray tube potentials, unshielded x-ray tubes, and long exposure times, many people suffered **inflammation**, erythema, and **desquamation** (peeling) to their skin. X-ray induced erythema was possibly the first observed biological response to irradiation. Radiation-induced skin erythema is analogous to that seen after extended exposure to the sun.

The skin is composed of an outer layer (**epidermis**), a middle layer of connective tissue (**dermis**), and a **subcutaneous** layer of fat and connective tissue. Accessory structures in the skin which originate in the dermis include the hair **follicle**s (sac), **sebaceous** (oily secretion) glands, sweat glands, and sensory receptors. All the skin's cell layers and accessory structures are involved in the response to irradiation. Figure 4–4 illustrates the skin and accessory structures.

The epidermis is composed of cell layers that consist of both mature nondividing cells (surface cells) and immature dividing cells (basal layer cells). The skin's surface regularly loses cells which must be replaced by the basal layer cells, at the rate of approximately 2% per day. The characteristics of the epidermis basal cells thus make the skin radiosensitive.

Within 1–2 days of a single dose of 100 to 1,000 rad, the skin may exhibit mild erythema. This initial erythema is followed by a more severe erythema in about 2 weeks. Prior to the introduction of radiation units, the **skin erythema dose (SED)** was used as a measure of the amount of radiation a person had received. Using data from people who were irradiated superficially with therapeutic x-rays, the skin erythema dose necessary to affect 50% of people so irradiated (**SED50**) is estimated to be approximately 600 rad

TABLE 4–3

ACUTE RADIATION SYNDROME SUMMARIZATION

Syndrome	Dose Range	Prodromal Effects	Manifest–Illness Effects	Survival without Treatment	Survival with Treatment
Hematologic	0.5–1.0 Gy (50–100 rads)	Mild	Slight decrease in blood cell count	Almost certain	Almost certain
	1.0–2.0 Gy (100–200 rads)	Mild to moderate	Early symptoms of bone marrow damage	Probably (>90%)	Almost certain
	2.0–3.5 Gy (200–350 rads)	Moderate	Moderate to severe bone marrow damage	Possible	Probable
	3.5–5.5 Gy (350–550 rads)	Moderate to severe	Severe bone marrow damage; slight intestinal damage	Death likely within 3–6 weeks	Possible
	5.5–8.0 Gy (550–800 rads)	Severe	Bone marrow pancytopenia and moderate intestinal damage	Death likely within 2–3 weeks	Possible if stem cell support or replacement is successful
	8.0–10.0 Gy (800–1,000 rads)	Severe	Combined gastrointestinal and bone marrow damage; hypotension	Death within 1.0–2.5 weeks	Death likely, but survival possible if stem cell support or replacement is successful.
Gastrointestinal	10.0–50.0 Gy (1,000–5,000 rads)	Severe prodromal symptoms, hematologic syndrome which overlaps with severe gastrointestinal damage; electrolyte imbalance; fatigue, gastrointestinal death		Death within 5–12 days	
Neurovascular	>50 Gy (5,000 rads)	Severe prodromal symptoms which overlap with CNS effects. Ataxia, severe edema, neurovascular damage, shock		Death within 2–5 days	

(Reproduced with permission from Bushberg, J. T., Seibert, J. A., Leidholt, E. M., and Boone, J. M. [2001]. The essential physics of medical imaging. [2nd ed.]. Philadelphia: Lippincott, Williams and Wilkins.

FIGURE 4–4
Skin and accessory structures

(6 Gy). Skin erythema is considered to follow a nonlinear, threshold dose-response relationship.

When the epidermis is exposed to moderate doses, it is permitted to heal by regenerating, which results in insignificant late changes. However, when exposed to high doses, late changes including atrophy, fibrosis, changes in pigmentation, ulcers, **necrosis** (tissue death) and cancer may occur.

Since hair follicles are actively growing tissue, they are radiosensitive. Moderate doses may cause temporary epilation or **alopecia** (hair loss), with high doses possibly resulting in permanent epilation.

Sebaceous and sweat glands are considered to be relatively **radioresistant**. Exposure to high doses causes glandular atrophy and fibrosis that results in minimal or no function.

Subjecting the skin to chronic irradiation may result in nonmalignant changes. The early radiologists developed hands and forearms that were calloused, discolored, and weathered in appearance. Their skin became tight and brittle, which led to cracking and flaking.

Because of the use of intensifying screens, beam-restricting devices, and radiation protection guidelines, today's doses from diagnostic radiographic and fluoroscopic exams pose minimal hazard in regards to the previously mentioned changes. Table 4–4 summarizes the effects of radiation on skin.

TABLE 4–4

RADIATION EFFECTS ON SKIN

Spectrum of Effects on Skin

Early Effects	Late Effects	Effect on Accessory Structures
Erythema	Atrophy	Epilation
Inflammation	Fibrosis	Destruction of sweat and
Dry Desquamation	Hyper/hypo pigmentation	sebaceous glands
Moist Desquamation	Ulceration	
	Necrosis	
	Cancer	

Dose/Time—Response Relationship

Dose	Radiation Dose Area	Exposure Internal	Type of Reaction or Damage
<1 Gy (100 rads)	Small	Short	No visible effect
2–6 Gy (200–600 rads)	Small	Short	Erythema in 1–2 days after exposure; persists until day 5–6; reappears on day 10–12; maximum on day 18–20; persists until day 30–40. Temporary hair 1oss if >3 Gy (300 rads)
6–10 Gy (600–1,000 rads)	Small	Short	More serious erythema caused by damage of basal cells. Symptoms appear earlier, are more intense, and healing is delayed.
15 Gy (1,500 rads) or 30 Gy (3,000 rads)	Small Small	Short ~4 weeks	Severe erythema, followed or by dry desquamation and delayed/ incomplete healing.
20–50 Gy (2,000–5,000 rads) or 40 Gy (4,000 rads)	Limited Limited	Short ~4 weeks	Intense erythema, acute radiation dermatitis with moist desquamation, edema, dermal hypoplasia, vascular damage and permanent hair loss, permanent tanning, destruction of sweat glands, vascular damage. If >5 Gy (5,000 rads) followed by ulceration/necrosis
20 Gy (2,000 rads)	Hands or other small area	Several years small daily doses (1–2 rads)	No early or intermediate changes. Late changes manifested by dry cracked skin, nails curled and cracked, intractable ulcers, possible cancerous changes.

(Reproduced with permission from Bushberg, J. T., Seibert, J. A., Leidholt, E. M., and Boone, J. M. [2001]. The essential physics of medical imaging. [2nd ed.]. Philadelphia: Lippincott, Williams and Wilkins.

Eyes

The lens of the eye contains radiosensitive cells that may be damaged or even destroyed by radiation. Because the body is not able to naturally remove damaged cells, they may accumulate to the point of causing cataracts. The formation of cataracts caused by radiation is termed **radiation cataractogenesis**. The extent of opacity and chance of occurrence are proportional to the dose.

Radiation-induced cataracts follow a threshold, nonlinear dose-response relationship. The threshold dose is thought to be approximately 200 rad (2 Gy). At doses of greater than 700 rad (7 Gy), all people irradiated will develop cataracts. The average latent period for cataract formation is approximately 15 years. High LET radiation has a high RBE for cataractogenesis by a factor of two or more. The efficiency of cataractogenesis is decreased by exposure to chronic doses.

Cataractogenesis was common among early radiation personnel and patients because of the extremely high doses from long exposure times and from exposures being produced by equipment which was poorly shielded. Cataractogenesis among today's radiation personnel is rare. It is nearly impossible for today's radiation personnel to reach the threshold dose. As the highest exposures to the eyes are received during fluoroscopic examinations, it is suggested that protective eyewear be worn while working in this high dose area. Protective lens shields should be provided to patients as long as their use does not interfere with the exam.

Gonads

Human gonads are extremely radiosensitive. Doses as low as 10 rad have caused observable responses. As gonads create germ cells that control fertility and heredity, their response to irradiation has been analyzed thoroughly.

Much of the data regarding gonadal irradiation response has come from animal experiments, and some has come from radiation therapy patients, radiation accident victims, and experiments on volunteer convicts.

The male testes and the female ovaries react differently to radiation because of variations in the way their germ cells progress from the stem cell phase to the mature cell. Figure 4–5 contrasts the life cycle of the **oogonia** with that of **spermatogonia**.

Both the ovaries and testes produce germ cells, but they have different rates and times in regard to the way they develop from **stem cell** to mature cell. The ovary stem cells, the oogonia, multiply only during fetal life. During midpregnancy, the oogonia in the fetus number about 7 million, and then start to decline in number throughout life. Conversely, the stem cells of the testes, the spermatogonia, are constantly reproducing.

Male   With the exception of the testes, the majority of the male gonad tissues are radioresistant. The testes contain the mature spermatozoa, which are nondividing, differentiated and radioresistant; they also include the immature spermatogonia, which are rapidly dividing, undifferentiated and

Male:

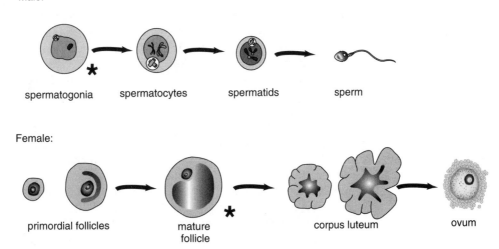

    spermatogonia   spermatocytes   spermatids   sperm

Female:

    primordial follicles   mature follicle   corpus luteum   ovum

* most radiosensitive

FIGURE 4–5
Oogonia versus spermatogonia life cycle

radiosensitive. The main effect of radiation on the male gonads is damage to and reduction in number of the spermatogonia, which ultimately leads to depletion of mature sperm, a process called **maturation depletion**. After testicular irradiation, there is a variable period of fertility caused by the radioresistance of the mature sperm. Depending on the dose, this period of fertility is followed by either temporary or permanent sterility. The cause of sterility is from the loss of immature spermatogonia that divide and replace the mature sperm lost from the testes. A dose of 200 to 250 rads produces temporary sterility, which may last up to 1 year. An acute dose of 500 to 600 rads causes permanent sterility.

Besides the possibility of sterility, another danger of irradiating the testes is the production of chromosomal abnormalities that may be passed on to future generations. The previously mentioned fertile period which occurs postexposure does not eliminate the chance of damage to the chromosomes in the functional spermatozoa. Also, chromosome damage to the immature spermatogonia cannot be ruled out.

Diagnostic radiology consists of acute low doses to patients and chronic low doses to personnel that present no danger regarding sterility. Nevertheless, these doses may cause chromosomal abnormalities that could result in mutations in future generations. Because of this, the testes should be shielded from unnecessary radiation whenever practical.

Female   The **ova,** which are enclosed within the follicles, are specified by size as small, intermediate and large. The radiosensitivity of the ova is as follows: most sensitive = intermediate follicles; most resistant = small follicles; and moderately sensitive = mature follicles. The ova do not continuously divide and replace those that are lost during menstruation. During ovulation, an ovum is released from a mature follicle. This is followed by either fertilization or menstruation. Following moderate doses of radiation to the ovaries, there is an initial period of fertility. This is caused by moderately resistant mature follicles being present which can release an ovum. The fertile period is succeeded by either temporary or permanent sterility. These sterilities are from the ova receiving damage in the radiosensitive intermediate follicles, which restricts their maturation and release.

A dose of 10 rads can restrain and retard menstruation. Sterility is a function of age, with the fetus and child being particularly radiosensitive. There is a decline in sensitivity until approximately age 30, when sensitivity begins to increase continually with age. Doses of 200 rads produce temporary sterility. An acute dose of approximately 500 to 600 rads will cause permanent sterility.

There is anxiety about the chance of genetic changes in the functional ova after being irradiated. Even though fertility recurs after low to moderate doses, it may be possible that the functional ova have suffered chromosomal damage which may produce abnormal offspring or even nonvisible mutations that will not become manifest until future generations.

Analogous to the male, because of the acute low doses received by patients and chronic low doses received by personnel, the likelihood of female sterility is minimal. However, as mentioned previously, the possibility of chromosomal damage cannot be excluded. Therefore, the ovaries should be shielded from radiation whenever practical.

HEMATOLOGIC EFFECTS

In the 1920s and 1930s, periodic blood examinations were used to monitor radiology personnel. Included in these exams were total cell and white cell differential counts. We now know that it takes a minimum whole-body dose of about 25 rads (250 mGy) to cause hematologic depression. Based on current radiation protection standards, we now know that these people were heavily irradiated. Periodic blood examinations for radiation protection purposes are not justified for current radiation protection programs.

Hemopoietic System

The hemopoietic system includes bone marrow, circulating blood, lymph nodes, spleen and thymus.

Included in bone marrow tissues are the parenchymal cells of the marrow, which include stem cells for cells in circulating blood and fat cells, and connective tissue **stroma** (support tissue). The two types of marrow found in adults are red and yellow. Red marrow, which includes a large number of stem cells along with fat cells, supplies mature functional cells to circulating blood. In the adult this marrow is located in the ribs, ends of long bones, vertebrae, sternum and skull. Yellow marrow, composed mostly of fat cells with few stem cells, does not actively deliver mature cells to the circulating blood. Because of its fat content, the yellow marrow is also known as fatty marrow.

In contrast to an adult, whose bone marrow is found in definite sites, there is uniform distribution of bone marrow in the fetus. Also, the majority of fetal bone marrow is red bone marrow.

The principal response of bone marrow to radiation is a decrease in the number of stem cells. Low radiation doses cause a slight decrease in stem cells followed by recovery within a few weeks postexposure. With moderate and high doses the depletion of stem cells is more intense, which leads either to a longer recovery period and/or less recovery. Less recovery is exhibited as an increased number of fat and connective tissue, and a permanent decrease of stem cells.

Even though all bone marrow stem cells are considered to be highly radiosensitive, the different cells display diversity as to their radiosensitivity. The most sensitive stem cells are the **erythroblasts** (precursor cells for red blood cells). Next in sensitivity are the **myelocytes** (precursors for white blood cells). The least sensitive stem cells are the **megakaryocytes** (precursors for platelets). Exposure to low radiation doses causes decreased stem cell numbers with rapid recovery. Moderate to high doses result in a more intense decrease in all cell lines accompanied by either slow or incomplete recovery of cell numbers.

Except for lymphocytes, cells in the circulating blood are considered radioresistant. Nevertheless, the circulating blood is an indication of how much damage the bone marrow has received. If there is a decrease in the number of stem cells in the marrow, there will be a coinciding decrease in the number of mature circulating cells.

The coincidence of damage to the bone marrow in the circulating blood cells depends on: a) the sensitivity of the various stem cells and b) the life span of each cell line. All circulating blood cells have a limited life span, which varies on the average from 1 day (**granulocytes**) to 120 days (erythrocytes).

Following radiation exposure, the lymphocytes are the first cells to be reduced (doses as low as 10 rads will decrease count). Second to respond are the neutrophils (doses of 50 rads are required to cause decrease). Last to respond are the platelets and red blood cells (doses greater than 50 rads are necessary). Figure 4–6 illustrates typical hematologic depression following bone marrow doses of (A) 100 rads and (B) 300 rads.

Low doses to the lymphocytes cause a minimal depression, which is followed by recovery and a return to pre-exposure lymphocyte values. After a moderate dose the lymphocyte counts approach zero within a few days, followed by full recovery within a few months postexposure.

Within one week postexposure, the neutrophil count falls to minimal values. Recovery begins shortly thereafter and within one month postexposure neutrophil counts approach normal.

For platelets and red blood cells, low doses in the moderate range have negligible effects. Higher doses in the moderate range cause obvious cell depression. For these cells, recovery begins four weeks postexposure, and usually is complete in a few months.

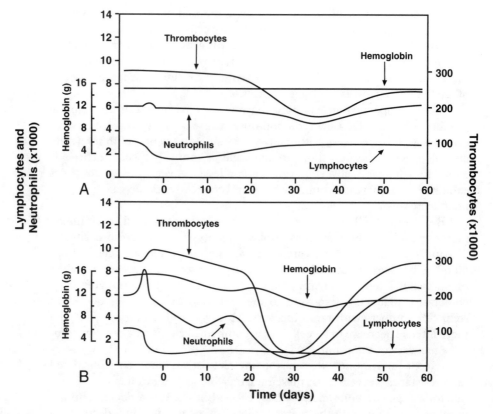

FIGURE 4-6
Hematologic depression bone marrow doses (Adapted from Andrews, G. [1980]. Medical management of accidental total body irradiation. In *The medical basis for radiation accident preparedness*, K. F., Hubner, & S. A., Fry, [Eds.]. New York: Elsevier.

If there is a decrease in the numbers of these various cells, there may be consequences throughout life. The body's defense mechanisms rely on neutrophils and lymphocytes in fighting off infections. If these cells are depleted, the person will be more vulnerable to infection. Platelets are required for blood clotting. If these cells are depleted, there is increased chance for hemorrhage. If there is depression of red blood cells, the result will be anemia.

Regarding decreased cell counts, diagnostic dose ranges present no significant dangers to the blood and blood-forming organs of patients or occupationally exposed personnel, although there have been chromosomal changes observed in this dose range.

CYTOGENETIC EFFECTS

Chromosomal damage can occur with low and high radiation doses. Although structural changes may be caused by either direct or indirect action, the majority of chromosomal damage occurs from indirect ionization. Damage results in breakage of the chromosome.

The structural changes to the chromosome that occur after irradiation are called **aberrations** (imperfection), **lesions** or **anomalies** (departure from normal). Chromosome aberrations that are caused by radiation can take place in both genetic and **somatic** cells. If chromosomal aberrations are not repaired before DNA synthesis, these aberrations may be transmitted during mitosis and meiosis.

Radiation-induced chromosomal damage that occurs before DNA synthesis is known as chromosomal aberration. If chromosomal repair does not happen before the S-phase of the cell cycle, a chromosomal break will be replicated. With chromosomal aberrations, both daughter cells inherit a damaged chromatid.

Radiation-induced chromosomal damage that occurs after DNA synthesis is called a chromatid aberration. While in the S-phase of the cell cycle, a chromosome duplicates itself. The two analogous chromosomes that are produced are known as sister chromatids. If only one pair of chromatids is damaged, only one daughter cell will be affected.

A chromatid aberration occurs after DNA synthesis. During the DNA synthesis phase, a chromosome duplicates itself. The two analogous chromosomes created are called sister chromatids. If only one pair of chromatids is injured, only one daughter cell will be affected.

The two primary types of chromosomal aberrations include single-break and double-break damage.

With single-break damage, a part of a chromosome arm is broken off. If the broken piece does not reattach itself, this is termed a terminal deletion; if it inverts and then reattaches itself, it is termed an inversion; if it attaches itself to a different chromosome, it is termed duplication.

In double-break damage, two portions of the chromosome are broken off. If the two broken pieces do not reattach themselves, this is termed interstitial deletion; if the broken pieces invert and reattach themselves to the chromosome arm, this is termed inversion; if one or both pieces attach to different a chromosome, this is termed duplication; with translocation, two chromosomes exchange pieces.

Factors that influence the repair of chromosomal aberrations include the stage of cell cycle and the type and location of the aberrations. The broken ends of chromosomes exhibit a strong force of cohesion. Recombination of chromosomes occurs in methods that produce aberrations such as **acentrics** (on the outside), **dicentrics** (having two centers), and rings. Figure 4–7 depicts common chromosomal aberrations and consequences.

The magnitude of total genetic damage that is transmitted by chromosomal aberrations depends upon the cell type, number and kind of genes damaged, and whether or not the aberration occurred in somatic or genetic cells.

If there is a change in a chromosome, there are corresponding changes in DNA. These changes in DNA cause the genetic information in the cell to be altered. This change in genetic information is called a mutation.

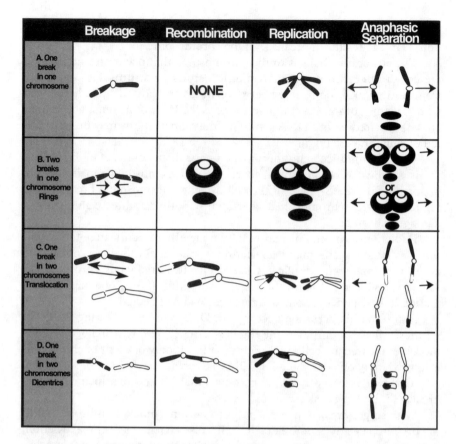

FIGURE 4–7

Common chromosomal aberrations and Consequences (Reproduced with permission from Bushberg, J. T., Seibert, J. A., Leidholt, E. M., and Boone, J. M. [2001]. *The essential physics of medical imaging.* [2nd ed.]. Philadelphia: Lippincott, Williams and Wilkins.

A **karyotype**, which is a chromosome map, is used for cytogenetic analysis of chromosomes. Photographs (photomicrographs) are taken and enlarged of the cell nucleus during metaphase which demonstrate each chromosome separately. The individual chromosomes are cut out and paired with their sister chromosomes on the map.

Consequences of chromosomal aberrations may not be able to be determined. If there is cell death, this is obviously a significant result. Numerous cell mutations go undetected and do not cause cell death. These discrete cell changes may be critical to humans. Somatic mutations have consequences for only that person. Genetic mutations can affect reproductive organs or the parent's **gametes**, which may affect future generations. It is presumed that genetic effects are cumulative.

Radiation cytogenetic data have shown that practically all types of chromosomal aberrations may be caused by radiation. The rate of production of aberrations is related to both total radiation dose and dose rate, and these appear to be nonthreshold. Chromosomal aberrations may be caused by both low and high radiation doses. Radiation effects on chromosomes appear to be nonspecific, and are not desirable.

KEY CONCEPTS

- Hematologic syndrome is exhibited by destruction of bone marrow caused by a reduction in production of red and white blood cells and platelets resulting from radiation exposure. Death may occur as a result of anemia and infection. Gastrointestinal syndrome is exhibited by nausea, vomiting, cramps, and diarrhea as a result of damage to the villi in the small intestine which leads to a lack of absorption. Dehydration and infection are the end results. Central nervous system syndrome is exhibited by nervousness, confusion, nausea, vomiting, loss of consciousness, and burning sensations of the skin which are the result of damage to blood vessels and increased intracranial pressure.

- Local tissue damage to the skin results in inflammation, redness and a breakdown of the tissue layers. Higher doses of radiation cause hair loss, changes in pigmentation, ulcers, tissue death and cancer. Radiation damage to the eyes results in cataracts. Tissue damage to the reproductive system as a result of radiation exposure may result in immature reproductive cell death leading to infertility and the possibility of genetic mutations in offspring.

- Radiation effects on the hematologic system reduce the number of stem cells produced by the bone marrow. A decrease in the number of white and red blood cells, as well as platelets, also occurs. Cytogenic effects as a result of radiation exposure result in damage and mutation of chromosomes.

Effects of Long-term Exposure to Radiation

KEY TERMS

Absolute risk model

Acute

Ankylosing
  spondylitis

BEIR

Benign

Carcinogenic

Carcinoma

Chronic

Doubling dose

Excess risk

Fibrosis

Follicular

Genetically
  significant dose
  (GSD)

Hypoxic

Leukemia

Loci

Lymphoid

Malignant

Myeloid

Neoplasm

Neuroblasts

Nonstochastic

Osteosarcoma

Papillary

Parenchymal

Progeny

Radiocarcinogenesis

Radium

Radon

Relative risk model

Stochastic

Turner's syndrome

Zygote

OBJECTIVES

Upon completion of this chapter, the reader should be able to:

- Discuss epidemiology
- Explain risk estimation models
- Examine radiation-induced malignancies
- Identify life span shortening
- Discuss genetic damage
- Explain irradiation of the fetus
- Analyze stochastic and nonstochastic effects

EPIDEMIOLOGY

Since the first documented case of radiation-induced **carcinoma** (growth or tumor) in 1902, it has been established that radiation is **carcinogenic** (cancer causing). Shortly after the discovery of x-rays, there were hundreds of cases of radiation induced skin cancers reported by radiology personnel. It is now known that radiation is also responsible for causing other types of malignancies.

While it has been well established that at high doses and high dose rates cancer is carcinogenic, this is not the case with the low doses that are associated with occupational exposures. Predominately through animal and statistical studies of human population groups, radiation has been associated with causing cancer. Risks to low levels of exposure are small, but exactly how small is debateable.

Incidence rates for radiation-induced cancer are determined by contrasting the expected occurrence in a control group (the general population) with the occurrence in an experimental group (the irradiated population). Risk factors are then calculated for the experimental group. The science which examines the incidence, distribution and control of disease in a population is termed epidemiology.

The following populations are used as sources of data on the incidence of radiation-induced cancer:

1. atomic bomb survivors
2. medically exposed patients
3. occupationally exposed personnel
4. populations who receive high natural background exposure

Table 5–1 lists sources of data on radiation exposure to humans.

Limitations on epidemiologic studies include the following:

• failure to control experimental group for other known carcinogens
• insufficient observation periods which permit full demonstration of cancers with long latent periods
• using improper control groups
• deficient or incorrect health records

Table 5–2 summarizes some of the main epidemiologic studies from which current dose-response estimates are derived.

Dose-Response Curves

Dose-response curves have been created by scientists who predict cancer risks in human populations that have been exposed to low levels of ionizing radiation. These dose-response curves are nonthreshold linear, linear quadratic, and quadratic. Figure 5–1 illustrates linear and linear quadratic dose-response curves.

Nonthreshold linear curves overestimate cancer incidence at lower doses from low LET radiation and accordingly are used for radiation protection guidelines when estimating the overall cancer risk from diagnostic and occupational exposures.

TABLE 5-1.

SOURCES OF DATA ON RADIATION EXPOSURE TO HUMANS

Atomic Bomb Detonation Exposures and Fallout
   Survivors
   Offspring of survivors

Medical Exposures
   Treatment of tinea capitis
   X-ray treatment of ankylosing spondylitis
   Prenatal diagnostic x-ray
   X-ray therapy for enlarged thymus glands
   Fluoroscopic guided pneumothorax for the treatment for
   tuberculosis
   Thorotrast (radioactive contrast material used in angiography
   1925–1945)
   Treatment of neoplastic diseases (e.g., breast cancer, Wilms' tumor,
   cancer of the cervix and leukemia)

Occupational Exposures
   Radium dial painters (1920s)
   Uranium miners and millers
   Nuclear dockyard workers
   Nuclear materials enrichment and processing workers
   Participants in nuclear weapons tests
   Construction workers
   Industrial photography workers
   Radioisotope production workers
   Reactor personnel
   Civil aviation and astronautic personnel
   Phosphate fertilizer industry workers
   Scientific researchers
   Diagnostic and therapeutic radiation medical personnel

Epidemiologic Comparisons of Areas with High-Background
   Radiation

(Reproduced with permission from Bushberg, J. T., Seibert, J. A., Leidholt, E. M., and Boone, J. M. [2001]. *The essential physics of medical imaging.* [2nd ed.]. Philadelphia: Lippincott, Williams and Wilkins.

Relative Versus Absolute Risk

The **relative** or multiplicative **risk model** explains how age at the time of radiation exposure may influence the cancer risk estimate. This model theorizes that following the latent period, the excess risk is a multiple of the natural age-specific cancer risk for the population being studied.

Another theory is the **absolute** or additive **risk model**. This model estimates a continual increase in risk that is independent of the spontaneous age specific cancer risk at the time of exposure. Figure 5–2 compares the relative and absolute risk models.

It is speculated that as a person ages, his cancer risk increases. Figure 5–3 demonstrates the effect of age on incidence.

TABLE 5–2

DOSE-RESPONSE EPIDEMIOLOGIC STUDIES

Summary of Major Epidemiologic Investigations That Form the Basis of Current Cancer Dose-Response Estimates in Human Populations*

Population & Exposure	Effects Observed	Strengths & Limitations
Atomic Bomb Survivors: A mortality study of approximately 120,000 residents of Hiroshima and Nagasaki(1950) among whom 93,000 were exposed at the time of the bombing. This group continues to be followed. The latest mortality assessment through 1987 has been completed. New dose estimates have been made recently which determined that neutrons were not, as previously thought, a significant component of the dose for either of the two cities. Mean organ doses have been calculated for twelve organs. Approximately 20,000 received doses between 1–5 cGy (1–5 rads) while ~1,100 received doses in excess of 2 Gy (200 rads).	A total of 483 excess cancers are thought to have been induced by radiation exposure resulting in an excess cancer mortality of 205. The natural incidence for this population would have predicted 2,670 cancers. The number of expected, observed and excess cancers by organ system is shown below. This data applies to the 41,000 persons who received 0.01 Sv (1 rem) or more. The mean dose was 0.23 Sv (23 rem). No statistically significant radiation-related increases were observed for uterus, cervix, pancreas, rectum, multiple myleloma, non-Hodgkins's lymphoma or chronic lymphocytic leukemia.	The analysis of the atom-bomb survivors is the single most important cohort which influence current radiation-induced cancer risk estimates. The. population is large and there is a wide range of doses from which it is possible to make determinations of the dose-response and the effects of modifying factors such as age on the induction of cancer. Data at high doses are limited; thus the analysis only included individuals in which the doses to internal organs were less than 4 Gy (400 rads). The survivors were not representative of a normal Japanese population in so far as many of the adult males were away on military service while those remaining presumably had some physical condition preventing them from active service. In addition, children and the elderly perished shortly after the detonation in greater numbers than did young adults, suggesting the possibility that the survivors may represent a hardier subset of the population.

Cancer Type	Expected	Incidence Data Observed	Excess
Breast	200	295	95
Lung	365	456	91
Stomach	1,222	1,307	85
Leukemia	67	141	74
Thyroid	94	132	38
Colon	194	223	29
Skin	76	98	22
Bladder	98	115	17
Liver	95	109	14
Esophagus	79	84	5
Brain & CNS	67	71	4
Bone & connective tissue	12	16	4
Non-Hodgkin's Lymphoma	72	76	4
Multiple myeloma	29	30	1
TOTALS	2,670	3,153	483

(continues)

TABLE 5-2 (continued)

DOSE-RESPONSE EPIDEMIOLOGIC STUDIES

Summary of Major Epidemiologic Investigations That Form the Basis of Current Cancer Dose-Response Estimates in Human Populations*

Population & Exposure	Effects Observed	Strengths & Limitations
Ankylosing Spondylitis: This cohort consists of approximately 14,000 patients treated with radiotherapy to the spine for ankylosing spondylitis throughout the United Kingdom between 1935–1954. Although individual dose records were not available, estimates were made which ranged from 1–25 Gy (100–2,500 rads) to the bone marrow and other various organs.	Mortality has been reported though 1982, at which point 727 cancer deaths had been reported. Excess leukemia rates were reported from which all absolute risk of 0.8 excess cases/cGy (rad)/year per million was estimated.	This group represents one of the largest bodies of data on radiation-induced leukemia in humans for which fairly good dose estimates exist. Control groups were suboptimal, however, and doses were largely unfractionated. In addition only cancer mortality (not incidence) was available for this cohort.
Postpartum Mastitis Study: This group consists of approximately 600 women, mostly between the ages of 20 and 40, treated with radiotherapy for postpartum acute mastitis in New York in the 1940s and 1950s for which ~1,200 nonexposed women with mastitis and siblings of both groups of women served as controls. Breast tissue doses ranged from 0.6–14 Gy (60–1,400 rad).	Forty-five year follow-up identified excess breast cancer in this population as compared with the general female population of New York.	A legitimate objection to using the data from this study to establish radiation-induced breast cancer risk factors is the uncertainty as to what effect the inflammatory changes associated with postpartum mastitis and the hormonal changes due to pregnancy have on the risk of breast cancer.
Radium Dial Painters: Young women who ingested radium (Ra-226 and Ra-228 with half-lives of approximately 1,600 and 7 years, respectively) while licking their brushes (containing luminous radium sulfate) to a sharp point during the application of luminous paint on dials and clocks in	Large increase in osteogenic sarcoma. Osteogenic sarcoma is a rare cancer (~5/106). Relative risk in the population was greater than 100 x's. No increase was seen below doses of 5 Gy (500 rad) but rose sharply thereafter.	One of only a few studies that analyzed the radiocarinogenic effectiveness of internal contamination with high LET radiation in humans.

(continues)

TABLE 5–2 (continued)

DOSE-RESPONSE EPIDEMIOLOGIC STUDIES

Summary of Major Epidemiological Investigations That Form the Basis of Current Cancer Dose-Response Estimates in Human Populations*

Population & Exposure	Effects Observed	Strengths & Limitations
the 1920s and 1930s. Over 800 followed.		
Thorotrast: Several populations were studied in which individuals were injected intravascularly with an x-ray contrast media, Thorotrast, used between 1925–1945. Thorotrast contains 25% by weight radioactive colloidal Th-232 dioxide. Th-232 is an alpha emitter with a half-life of approximately 14 billion years.	Particles were deposited in the reticuloendothial systems. Noted increase in number of liver cancers, particularly angiosarcomas, bile duct carcinomas, and hepatic cell carcinomas. Evaluation of the data resulted in estimates of alpha radiation-induced liver cancer risk of approximately $300/10^4$ per Gy (100 rad) which appears to be linear with dose.	Dose estimates are fairly good. However, the extent to which the chemical toxicity of the Thorotrast may have influenced the risk is not known.

*Adapted from the 1990 National Academy of Sciences/National Research Council Committee on the Biological Effects of Ionizing Radiation report entitled, *The Health Effects of Exposure to Low Levels of Ionizing Radiation (BEIR V).*

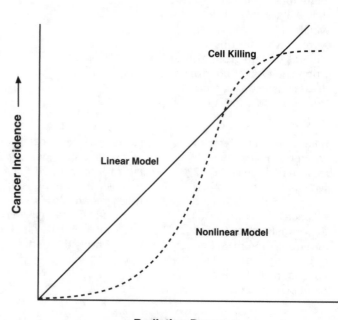

FIGURE 5–1

Linear and linear quadratic dose-response models

FIGURE 5–2 Relative and absolute risk models

Risk Expression   Relative risk is one method of expressing the risk from radiation to an exposed population. This risk is the ratio of cancer incidence in an exposed population to that of an unexposed population. It can be used when there is no exact knowledge of radiation dose.

$$\text{The formula for relative risk} = \frac{\text{observed cases}}{\text{expected cases}}$$

EXAMPLE

A relative risk of 1.5 would indicate a 50% increase in the irradiated group as compared with the non-irradiated group.

Relative risk rates range from 1 to 10, with 1 representing no risk at all. Most reports for the observed late effects in humans are in the range from 1 to 2.

FIGURE 5–3

Effect of age on cancer incidence

EXAMPLE

A study of radiation-induced **leukemia** (cancer of blood forming cells in bone marrow) was performed after diagnostic levels of radiation. 400 cases were observed in 150,000 people irradiated. The normal incidence of leukemia is 120 cases per 100,000. If the normal incidence were presumed to occur in a non-irradiated population, what is the relative risk of radiation-induced leukemia?

Correct response: Relative risk $= \dfrac{\text{observed cases}}{\text{expected cases}}$

$\dfrac{400}{150,000} = 0.003 \qquad \dfrac{120}{100,000} = 0.0012$

Relative risk $= \dfrac{0.003}{0.0012} = 2.5$

Absolute risk states risk in terms of number of cases/10^6 persons/rad/year. This type of risk assumes a linear dose-response relationship. Absolute risk can be determined when at least two different dose levels are known.

EXAMPLE

Absolute risk for radiation-induced breast cancer is presumed to be six cases/10^6 persons/rad/yr at a 15 year at-risk period. If 10,000 women receive 1 rad during mammography, what would be the total number of cancers expected to be produced?

Correct response:

(6 cases/10^6 persons/rad/yr)(10^4 persons)(1 rad)(15 yr) = 0.9

$$\frac{6}{1,000,000} = 0.000006$$

$0.000006 \times 10^4 \times 1 \times 15 = 0.9$

Excess risk is another way to express risk. This risk is described as the number of excess cases observed compared with the expected spontaneous occurrence. When scientists can observe the number of cases in the irradiated population and compare this with the number that is normally expected, excess risk can be determined.

The formula for excess risk = observed cases – expected cases.

EXAMPLE

13 cases of skin cancer were detected in a population of 2,000 radiologists. The incidence for the general population is 0.5/100,000. How many excess skin cancers were produced in the radiologist population?

Correct response:

excess cases = observed cases – expected cases =
13 - 0.000005 = ~12.9

The relative and absolute risk models are most often used for expressing risk. The **BEIR** Committee (Committee on the Biological Effects of Ionizing Radiation), which is associated with the National Academy of Sciences, used the relative risk model.

Table 5–3 lists the overall risk and relative probabilities of radiation-induced cancer mortality in various organs for different age groups.

TABLE 5-3

RISK AND RELATIVE PROBABILITIES OF CANCER FOR DIFFERENT AGES

Overall Risk and Relative Probabilities of Radiation-Induced Cancer Mortality in Various Organs for Different Age Groups[a]

Organ	Age Group		
	0–19 Years	0–90 Years	20–64 Years
Stomach	0.243	0.266	0.303
Lung	0.245	0.203	0.144
Bone Marrow	0.054	0.091	0.137
Bladder	0.030	0.054	0.081
Colon	0.218	0.154	0.078
Esophagus	0.023	0.040	0.062
Ovary[b]	0.011 (0.22)	0.017 (0.034)	0.024 (0.048)
Breast[b]	0.030 (0.60)	0.025 (0.05)	0.021 (0.042)
Remainder	0.150	0.150	0.150
Total	1.000	1.000	1.000
Risk 10^{-2}/Sv (10^{-4}/rem)	12	5.4	4

[a]Adapted from ICRP Report No. 60
[b]This table represents the ICRP's risk coefficients for a working population that is assumed to be half women and half men. The risks for ovaries and breasts for women alone (in parentheses) is therefore twice this risk. No coefficient was specifically given for testis, which is included in the remainder risk coefficient.

RADIATION-INDUCED MALIGNANCIES

Many biological effects that are radiation-induced are discovered shortly after exposure. However, ionizing radiation is capable of causing damage that does not manifest itself for years or even decades.

Radiation-induced malignancies include leukemia, skin carcinoma, thyroid cancer, breast cancer, **osteosarcoma** (bone cancer) and lung cancer.

Leukemia

The first incidence of radiation-induced leukemia was in 1911. Since then, radiation has been associated with leukemia in studies of adult population groups that include atomic bomb survivors, **ankylosing spondylitis** (immobility of the vertebrae) patients who were treated with radiation, and radiologists.

Data from the atomic bomb survivors from Hiroshima and Nagasaki demonstrate a substantial increase in the incidence of leukemia when comparing the exposed with the unexposed population. From 1950–1956, 64 out of 117 new cases of leukemia were associated with radiation. In Hiroshima 61 leukemia deaths were observed as compared with the expected incidence of 12.

$$\text{Relative risk} = \frac{\text{observed cases}}{\text{expected cases}} = \frac{61}{12} = 5.08$$

In Nagasaki 20 leukemia deaths were observed as compared with the expected incidence of 7.

$$\text{Relative risk} = \frac{20}{7} = 2.85$$

Increased rates of leukemia were observed at Hiroshima at low doses (20–50 rads), but these increases were not seen at Nagasaki. These differences in incidence are attributed to the different types of radiation that each city was exposed to. Approximately 90% of the dose at Nagasaki was from x-rays, whereas at Hiroshima approximately half the dose was from x-rays and half was from neutrons. Neutrons have a higher RBE than x-rays, and are thus more biologically damaging.

From 1935 to 1944, approximately 15,000 patients with ankylosing spondylitis were treated with radiation in Great Britain. These patients received both acute and fractionated doses to the pelvis and spine that ranged from 100 to 2,000 R. A fractionated dose is one that is given in smaller quantities over a period of time.

In a two-year follow-up study, seven cases of leukemia were documented as compared with the expected incidence of one. In patients who received doses over 2,000 R, there was an increased incidence of leukemia of over 100%.

The early radiologists make up another group where radiation is considered to cause leukemia. A study in the United States of 425 radiologists who died between 1948 and 1961 shows an incidence of 12 cases of leukemia as compared with an expected incidence of 4.

A British study of radiologists who entered practice after 1921 demonstrated no excess in leukemia. This study is of significance, since it contradicts the American radiologist study.

Currently, the incidence of leukemia among American radiologists is not higher than other physician specialties. There is no evidence of radiation-induced leukemia in studies of American radiographers.

With the incidence of leukemia in the U.S. at approximately 70/10,000, it is considered a rare disease. Even so, leukemia is one of the most frequently observed radiation-induced cancers. It is responsible for approximately one-sixth of the fatalities from **radiocarcinogenesis**. Leukemia can be **acute** (rapid and severe) or **chronic** (slow and progressive). It may be either **lymphoid** (in lymph tissue) or myeloid (in marrow). Excluding chronic lymphocytic leukemia, irradiated human population groups and animals who have been irradiated experimentally show increases in all forms of leukemia.

Age at the time of irradiation influences the incidence of leukemia. The incidence of radiation-induced leukemia decreases with age, as does the interval of increased risk. Figure 5–4 illustrates the effect of age at time of exposure on incidence of leukemia.

Radiation-induced leukemia is judged to be linear, nonthreshold, and has a latent period of 4–7 years with an at-risk period of 15–20 years.

The BEIR committee suggests a relative risk, nonlinear dose-response relationship for leukemia. It estimates the excess lifetime risk to be 10/10,000 (0.1%) after an exposure of 10 rads (0.1 Gy).

Skin Carcinoma

Within 15 years of the discovery of x-rays, hundreds of cases of skin carcinoma were reported by radiology personnel. Also occurring during the early years of radiation is another source of data from people who were treated with radiation for acne and ringworm and developed skin cancer years later.

Even though radiation-induced skin carcinomas cannot be distinguished from skin carcinomas caused by other methods, there is enough proof to connect radiation with skin cancer. The previously mentioned

FIGURE 5–4

Effect of age at time of exposure on incidence of leukemia (From Ichuimaru et al., Incidence of leukemia in atomic bomb survivors, Hiroshima and Nagasaki, 1950–1971, by radiation dose years after exposure, age, and type of leukemia, *Technical Report RERF* 10-76, Radiation Effects Research Foundation, Hiroshima, 1976) groups of people were exposed to unfiltered low kV x-rays which deliver very high doses to the superficial skin layers. These incidents prompted radiation safety regulations to be established.

Radiation-induced skin carcinoma follows a threshold dose-response relationship, and has a latent period of 5–10 years. In the 500 to 2,000 rad range, the relative risk for skin cancer is 4 to 1. With doses in the 6,000 to 10,000 rad range, the relative risk is 27 to 1. Radiation-induced skin carcinomas are not present in current radiology personnel.

Thyroid Cancer

The 1920s and 1930s saw infants with thymic enlargement being treated with radiotherapy. Doses to the thyroid were in the 120 to 6,000 R range. In a study of approximately 3,000 infants who received on average 120 rads, there were 24 observed cases of thyroid cancer. The expected incidence was 0.24 cases. This resulted in a hundredfold increase in thyroid cancer incidence. In a control group composed of approximately 5,000 unexposed infants, no cases of thyroid cancer were demonstrated. Another source of data comes from the offspring of the Marshall Islanders who were accidentally exposed to fallout radiation from nuclear bomb testing. These children in later years demonstrated an increased incidence of all types of thyroid disease, which included **benign** (nonprogressive) and **malignant** (progressive) tumors.

Studies of individuals who were children at the time of the atomic bombings in Nagasaki and Hiroshima have also shown increased incidences of thyroid cancer.

Thyroid cancer is responsible for approximately 12% of the deaths attributed to radiation-induced malignancies. Females have approximately a 3–5 times greater risk for radiation-induced thyroid cancer than males, because of hormonal influences on thyroid function.

Radiation-induced thyroid cancers are either **papillary** (nipple-like protrusion) or **follicular** (cavity), which are usually benign and slow growing, with a mortality rate of about 5%. The latent period for benign nodules is 5–35 years, and for malignant nodules 10–35 years. Internal irradiations from radionuclides such as iodine-131 have not been proven to cause thyroid cancer. The dose-response relationships for thyroid cancers are linear, nonthreshold.

Breast Cancer

The United States' breast cancer incidence for women is approximately 85/100,000 year or 1 in 11 lifetime. With low LET radiation, breast cancer risk seems to be age dependent. The risk for the 15-year old age group (30/10,000 or 0.3% year) is approximately 50 times higher after an exposure of 10 rads (0.1 Gy) than in women over the age of 55. According to the BEIR report, risk estimates for women in the 25, 35, and 45–year old age groups are 0.05, 0.04 and 0.02%, respectively. Breast cancer data appear to fit a linear dose-response relationship. In order to double the natural incidence of breast cancer, a dose of approximately 80 rads (0.8 Gy) is necessary. According to data from current acute and chronic exposure studies, it seems that fractionating the dose reduces the risk of low LET radiation-induced breast cancer. The latent period varies from 10–40 years. Absolute risk is estimated to be approximately six cases/10^6 persons/rad/year.

Because of recent improvements in mammography, there have been significant reductions in breast radiation doses. Even though theoretically mammography could increase the risk of breast cancer, studies have not demonstrated that the low doses received during a mammogram increase the risk of breast cancer.

Osteosarcoma

Bone cancers were noted in the watch-dial painters in the early 1920s. These people applied luminescent **radium** on watch hands and faces. In order to get a fine tip on their brush, they would put the tip in their mouth and pull it out. Radium was ingested by these workers and, being metabolically similar to calcium, was deposited in bone. Radium has a half-life of 1,620 years, meaning that it continued to be deposited at full strength throughout the person's lifetime. In a 1978 study of approximately 1,500 women employed in the industry before 1930, there were 61 cases of bone cancer, and 21 cases of sinus and mastoid carcinomas. Data analysis of the painters indicated an overall relative risk of 122:1. The absolute risk is 0.11 cases/10^6 persons/rad/yr. Osteosarcoma follows a linear quadratic dose-response relationship.

Lung Cancer

Increased incidences of lung cancer have been demonstrated in miners of uranium and pitchblende. Data from studies of the German pitchblende miners revealed that approximately 50% of them died from lung carcinoma. The general population had negligible incidences of lung cancer. These carcinomas were attributed to the radiation exposure received from **radon** in the mines.

A study of uranium miners in the Colorado plateau from 1950 to 1967 demonstrated 62 cases of lung cancer, which is 6 times the expected number. One of the decay products of uranium is the gas radon. The miners would inhale the radon, which would be deposited in their lungs. It would then decay into a stable isotope of lead. During decay, alpha-particles, which are high LET and therefore high RBE, were released and resulted in high local doses.

Dose-response relationships for radiation-induced lung cancer are linear nonthreshold. Based on data from over 4,000 uranium miners, an absolute risk of 1.3 cases/10^6 persons/rad/yr has been calculated.

Table 5–4 lists the spontaneous incidence and sensitivity of various tissues to radiation-induced cancer.

TABLE 5-4

SPONTANEOUS INCIDENCE AND SENSITIVITY OF TISSUES TO CANCER

Spontaneous Incidence and Sensitivity of Various Tissues to Radiation-induced Cancera

Site or Type of Cancer	Spontaneous Incidence	Radiation Sensitivity
Most Frequent Radiation-induced Cancers		
Female breast	Very high	High
Thyroid	Low	Very high, especially in females
Lung (bronchus)	Very high	Moderate
Leukemia	Moderate	Very high
Alimentary tract	High	Moderate to low
Less Frequent Radiation-induced Cancers		
Pharynx	Low	Moderate
Liver and biliary tract	Low	Moderate
Pancreas	Moderate	Moderate
Lymphomas	Moderate	Moderate
Kidney and bladder	Moderate	Low
Brain and nervous system	Low	Low
Salivary glands	Very low	Low
Bone	Very low	Low
Skin	High	Low
Magnitude of Radiation Risk Uncertain		
Larynx	Moderate	Low
Nasal sinuses	Very low	Low
Parathyroid	Very low	Low
Ovary	Moderate	Low
Connective tissue	Very low	Low

(continues)

TABLE 5-4 (continued)

SPONTANEOUS INCIDENCE AND SENSITIVITY OF TISSUES TO CANCER		
Spontaneous Incidence and Sensitivity of Various Tissues to Radiation-induced Cancera		
Site or Type of Cancer	**Spontaneous Incidence**	**Radiation Sensitivity**
Radiation Risk Not Demonstrated		
Prostate	Very high	Absent?
Uterus and cervix	Very high	Absent?
Testis	Low	Absent?
Mesothelium	Very low	Absent?
Chronic lymphatic leukemia	Low	Absent?

aAdapted from Committee on Radiological Units, Standards and Protection: *Medical Radiation: A Guide to Good Practice*. Chicago: American College of Radiology, 1985.

LIFE SPAN SHORTENING

Data from studies of animals that received acute and chronic radiation indicate that animals that were chronically irradiated died younger than animals that were not irradiated. Examinations of the dead animals showed a decreased number of **parenchymal** (essential, life-sustaining) cells and blood vessels along with increases in connective tissue in organs. These are suggestions of an aging process. This is regarded as radiation-induced aging. The correlation between life span shortening and dose is linear, non-threshold.

Nonspecific life span shortening caused by radiation has been reported in humans, although it appears to be caused by other radiation-induced effects, for example, leukemia, especially in the low dose ranges.

Radiologists from the 1930s were found to die 5 years younger than a control group of other doctors. A repeat study in the 1960s showed that this difference in death had shrunk to zero. This may be credited to improved radiation protection guidelines.

Life span shortening has not been observed in atomic bomb survivors, watch-dial painters or x-ray patients. Data from radiographers in WW II also showed no such effects.

GENETIC DAMAGE

Evidence of the ability of ionizing radiation to produce genetic damage was first acquired from a comprehensive study of fruit flies done in 1927 by

Herman Muller. Muller exposed male and female fruit flies to various doses of radiation, observed lethality and changes in appearance in offspring of irradiated parents, and compared these results with the unirradiated control group.

Muller's study concluded that:

1. No new or unique mutations are produced by radiation. Radiation simply increased the number of mutations found spontaneously in nature.
2. In the dose range of 25–400 R, the frequency of mutations was linear with dose. No threshold was observed. Equal dose increases were followed by an equal number of increases in the number of mutations. The observed effects were considered linear nonthreshold.
3. The majority of radiation-induced mutations were recessive. Both parents would have to carry the gene for an effect to be observed in offspring.
4. There were no dose rate or dose fractionation effects. This implies that mutations were single-hit and cumulative.

An ongoing experiment with irradiating mice was started by Russell in 1946. Data from this study demonstrate that:

1. Radiation is a powerful mutagenic agent.
2. The majority of mutations are unhealthy to the organism.
3. There are no unique mutations produced by radiation.
4. Radiation-induced genetic damage can occur as the result of a single mutation.

Initially, it was hypothesized that genetic effects were thought to be the most serious biological outcome from ionizing radiation. For the doses used in occupational and medical exposure, risks are small when compared with the spontaneous incidence of genetic aberrations, and are second to its carcinogenic capability.

Epidemiologic studies have not demonstrated radiation-induced genetic effects, although mutations of human cells in culture have been shown. For given exposures, mutation rates found in the offspring of irradiated humans are much lower than those previously identified in insect populations.

The largest human population studied is that of atomic bomb survivors and their offspring. A blood screening of 27,000 children of atomic bomb survivors for 28 specific protein **loci** demonstrated only 2 mutations that might be caused by radiation exposure of their parents.

Previous studies of atomic bomb survivors' **progeny** (offspring) were performed to determine if exposure to radiation caused an increase in sex-linked genes that would result in increased prenatal death of males or alteration of the gender birth ratio. The results of this study were negative. Irradiation to human testes has demonstrated an increase in incidence of translocations, although no additional chromosomal aberrations in atomic bomb survivors' progeny have been detected.

In order to evaluate the genetic influence of low doses to the whole population, the term **genetically significant dose (GSD)** is used. The GSD is an average calculated from the gonadal dose received by the entire population. It takes into account the expected contribution of these people to children in future generations. The GSD assumes that this dose, if received by every member of the population, would have the identical genetic effect as the doses that are received by those people who are actually exposed to radiation. When determining the GSD, the equivalent dose to the gonads of each irradiated person is weighted for the number of offspring expected for a person of that sex and age.

The annual GSD from all radiation sources is approximately 130 mrem (1.3 mSv). The single largest contribution, approximately 102 mrem (1.02 mSv) or 78%, comes from natural background radiation, primarily from cosmic rays, terrestrial exposure, and radionuclides within the body. The contribution from radon is minimal, approximately 10 mrem (100 mSv).

Technological sources contribute to the GSD predominately in the form of medical exposures, approximately 20 mrem (200 mSv) or 15%. About two-thirds of this is attributable to irradiation of females and one-third to males. Exposure is higher for females because of the location of the ovaries within the pelvis, which places them in the primary beam during radiographs of the abdomen and pelvis. Table 5–5 lists the annual GSD in the U.S. population.

Data from experiments have given rise to the concept of the **doubling** dose. This is the dose of radiation required per generation to double the spontaneous mutation rate. The spontaneous mutation rate is approximately 6%.

EXAMPLE

If 5% of the progeny in each generation have mutations, the doubling dose would eventually cause 10% mutations.

In data extrapolated from animal studies, the doubling dose for humans is estimated to be in the range of 50 to 250 rads (0.5 and 2.5 Gy) for each generation. A dose range is given because of the differences in frequency of mutations that are observed with chronic and acute exposure. The doubling dose for chronic exposure tends to be toward the higher dose range, and for acute exposure is toward the lower end of the range.

Essentially, if each individual of childbearing potential in the entire population were exposed to a gonadal dose of 50–250 R for many generations, there would eventually be twice the number of mutations in their progeny.

It is estimated by the BEIR Committee that an exposure of 1 rad (1 cGy) given to the present generation would cause 6–65 additional genetic disorders per million births in the succeeding generation. If the population is continually exposed to an increased dose of 1 rad for each generation, equilibrium is created between the initiation of new genetic disorders and the loss of remaining ones. An additional 100 genetic disorders would be expected in the population at equilibrium, mostly from clinically mild

TABLE 5-5

ANNUAL GSD IN THE UNITED STATES POPULATION		
Source	**Contribution to GSD (mrem)**	**% of total**
Natural Sources		
Radionuclides in body	36	
Terrestrial	28	
Cosmic	27	
Radon	10	
Cosmogenic	1	
Subtotal	102	78
Technological Sources		
Diagnostic x-rays	20	
Nuclear medicine	2	
Consumer products	5	
Other	<1	
Subtotal	~28	22
Total	130	100

autosomal dominant mutations. Chromosomal damage and recessive mutations contribute only minimally to the equilibrium rate. Even though some cancers are genetic in origin, it has not been proven that radiation has the capability to influence the inheritance of cancer susceptibility. Table 5–6 lists estimates of excess genetic effects following doses of 1 rad per generation.

The human gene pool has the ability to absorb large amounts of radiation damage without seriously affecting the population. Variations in natural background exposure do not contribute greatly to the population's genetic risk.

EXAMPLE

A dose of 10 rads (10 cGy) only produces approximately 200 additional genetic disorders/million live births in the first generation (0.002%/rad). The normal incidence of genetic disorders is approximately 1 in 20 or 5%. Therefore, the 10 rad (10 cGy) dose would cause an increase in the spontaneous rate of genetic disorders of less than 0.4%.

TABLE 5-6

ESTIMATES OF EXCESS GENETIC EFFECTS FOLLOWING DOSES OF 1 RAD PER GENERATION[a,b]

Type of Disorder	Current Incidence per 10⁶ Live–born Offspring	Additional Cases per 10⁶ Live–born Offspring per 10 mSv per Generation	
		First Generation	Equilibrium
Autosomal dominant[c]			
Clinically severe	2,500	5–20	25
Clinically mild	7,500[d]	1–15	75
X–linked	400	<1	<5
Recessive	2,500	<1	VSI
Chromosomal			
Unbalanced translocations	600[e]	<5	VLI
Trisomies	3,800[f]	<1	<1
Congenital abnormalities	20,000–30,000	10	10–100
Other disorders of complex etiology[g]			
Heart disease	600,000	NE	NE
Cancer	300,000	NE	NE
Selected others	300,000	NE	NE

[a]Adapted from the 1990 National Academy of Sciences/National Research Council Committee on the Biological Effects of Ionizing Radiation report entitled, *The Health Effects of Exposure to Low Levels of Ionizing Radiation (BEIR V).*

[b]Risks pertain to average population exposure of 10 mSv per generation to a population with the spontaneous genetic burden in humans and a doubling dose for chronic exposure of 1 Sv (100 rem). VSI = very slow increase; VLI = very little increase; NE = not estimated.

[c]"Clinically severe" assumes that survival and reproduction are reduced by 20–80% relative to normal. "Clinically mild" assumes that survival and reproduction are reduced by 1 to 20% relative to normal.

[d]Obtained by subtracting an estimated 2,500 clinically severe dominant traits from an estimated total incidence of dominant traits of 10,000.

[e]Estimated frequency from UNSCEAR Reports (1982 and 1986).

[f]Most frequent result of chromosomal nondisjunction among liveborn children. Estimated frequency from UNSCEAR (1982 and 1986).

[g]Lifetime prevalence estimates may vary according to diagnostic criteria and other factors. The values given for heart disease and cancer are round-numbered approximations for all varieties of the diseases. With regard to heart disease, no implication is made that any form of heart disease is caused by radiation among exposed individuals. The effect, if any, results from mutations that may be induced by radiation and expressed in later generations, which contribute, along with other genes, to the genetic component of susceptibility. This is analogous to environmental risk factors that contribute to the environmental component of susceptibility. The magnitude of the genetic component in susceptibility to heart disease and other disorders with complex etiologies is unknown.

The doses associated with diagnostic and occupational radiation exposures, even though increasing the dose to the gonads of those irradiated, would not be anticipated to cause any significant risk to their offspring.

IRRADIATION OF THE FETUS

A developing organism is a highly dynamic system that is characterized by rapid cell proliferation, migration, and differentiation. Based upon the law of Bergonie and Tribondeau, we know that the developing embryo is very radiosensitive. The embryo's response to irradiation depends upon the following factors:

- total dose
- rate of dose
- quality of radiation
- stage of development

The combination of these factors determines the type and extent of damage that can occur. The principal effects of irradiation to the fetus include:

- prenatal or neonatal death
- congenital abnormalities
- growth impairment
- reduced intelligence
- genetic abnormalities
- cancer induction

A fetus undergoes three stages of development: pre-implantation, major organogenesis, and fetal or growth stage. Each of these stages is distinguished by differing responses to irradiation, which are caused by the relative radiosensitivity of the tissues at the time of exposure.

Data on the effects of irradiation in utero have been obtained from the offspring of the atomic bomb survivors and children whose mothers received diagnostic and therapeutic irradiation during pregnancy. Microcephaly and mental and growth retardation were the principal effects that were seen. Abnormalities of the eyes, genitals and skeleton occured less often.

Children from Hiroshima and Nagasaki who were irradiated in utero between the 8- to 25–week postconception period demonstrated lower IQ scores than did the non-irradiated children. These effects were not observed in those children who were exposed before the 8th week or after the 25th week. This decrease in IQ was dependent on dose, and had a presumed threshold below 25 rads (250 mGy). These data demonstrated the greatest sensitivity for radiation-induced mental retardation is between the 8th and 25th week during which the risk is about 1/250 or 0.4% per 100 rad to the fetus.

Children who were irradiated in utero at the time of the atomic bomb detonation were observed to have microcephaly. The normal incidence of microencephaly is approximately 3%. In the dose range of 10–49 rads

(100–490 mGy) the incidence of microcephaly was approximately 19% and 6% for the 1st and 2nd trimesters, respectively. At doses greater than 100 rads (1 Gy) the microcephaly incidence jumped to approximately 83% and 42% for exposures in the 1st and 2nd trimesters, respectively.

The predominant scientific opinion is that there are thresholds for the majority of congenital abnormalities. Compared with the spontaneous incidence of congenital anomalies, which is approximately 4–6%, doses less than 10 rads (100 mGy) carry negligible risk. At doses below this threshold, therapeutic abortions would not normally be warranted. Radiation was once used to induce therapeutic abortion in cases where surgery was considered to be unwise. The normal treatment was 350–500 rads (3.5–5 Gy) given over 2 days, which usually resulted in fetal death within 1 month. In current diagnostic procedures, fetal irradiation rarely exceeds 5 rads (50 mGy). This dose range has not demonstrated any significant risk for congenital malformation or retarded growth.

Pre-implantation Stage

This stage originates with the joining of the sperm and egg, and continues through day 9 when the **zygote** becomes deposited in the intrauterine wall. During this stage, the fertilized ovum is repeatedly dividing to form a ball of highly undifferentiated cells.

Radiation damage during this stage can cause prenatal death. The incidence of congenital abnormalities is low during this stage, although not completely absent. Embryos that survive display the all-or-nothing response. If prenatal death does not happen, visible signs of abnormalities are unlikely, as injured cells are repaired or replaced.

Factors that contribute to the cell's resistance to radiation-induced abnormalities include their capability of repair, undifferentiation, and the **hypoxic** (poorly oxygenated) state of the embryo. During the first few cell divisions, the cells are undifferentiated and are not pre-determined for a specific organ system. Nevertheless, if there is chromosomal damage at this point, it may be passed on and expressed at a later time. Once cells are no longer indeterminate, losing even a few cells may cause anomalies, retarded growth, or prenatal death. The most critical times of exposure are at 12 hours postconception, when the two pronuclei fuse to the one-cell stage, and at 30 and 60 hours, which is when the first two division take place.

Radiation-induced chromosomal aberrations at the one-cell stage may lead to a loss of a chromosome in future cell divisions that would be similar throughout the embryo. At this early stage, the majority of chromosomal loss is fatal. If there is a loss of a sex chromosome in the female, this may cause **Turner's syndrome**. This syndrome is an endocrine disorder caused by failure of the ovaries to respond to pituitary hormone stimulation.

Data obtained from animal experiments show an increase in the spontaneous abortion rate after doses of 5–10 rads (50–100 mGy) given during the pre-implantation stage. Following implantation, doses of at least 25 rads (250 mGy) are necessary to cause prenatal death. The natural occurrence of spontaneous abortion is approximately 25–50%.

Major Organogenesis The incidence of congenital abnormalities are more frequent during the period of major organogenesis, which is the 2nd to 8th week after conception. The differentiation of cells to form specific organ systems occurs on a specific gestational day.

EXAMPLE

The stem cells of the CNS, the **neuroblasts**, appear on the 18th gestational day, the forebrain and eyes start to form on the 20th day, and primitive germ cells appear on the 21st day.

Organ systems are not at equal risk during the entire stage of major organogenesis. The critical period for probability of a malformation occurs when there is irradiation during the period of peak differentiation of that system. Some aberrations have demonstrated more than one critical period.

EXAMPLE

In mice, cataractogenesis has three critical periods.

Figure 5–5 demonstrates the critical periods for radiation-induced birth defects in humans.

FIGURE 5–5
Critical periods for radiation-induced birth defects (Data from Dekaban, A. S. Abnormalities in children exposed to x-irradiation during various stages of gestation: tentative timetable of radiation injury to human fetus. *J Nucl Med* 1968; 9: 471–477)

The CNS is the only organ system that has shown a relationship between congenital anomalies and low LET radiation at doses less than 25 rads (250 mGy). Because of the depletion of cells, embryos that are irradiated early in organogenesis show the greatest intrauterine retardation of growth. Hiroshima atomic bomb survivors who received in utero exposures greater than 10 rads (100 mGy) showed increased incidences of microcephaly.

Overall, radiation-induced teratogenic effects are less frequent in humans than in animals. This is because of the smaller fraction of the gestational period in which humans are in organogenesis (e.g., approximately 1/15 for humans vs. 1/3 for mice). However, the development of the CNS takes place over a much longer gestational period in humans than in animals, so it is more likely to be a target for radiation-induced injury. The CNS is not fully developed until approximately age 12 years. All cases of human irradiation in utero which resulted in gross malformations have been accompanied by CNS aberrations and/or retarded growth.

Each organ is unique in how it responds to the induction of radiation-induced malformations. Factors such as gestational age, radiation quality/quantity/dose rate, oxygen tension and type of cell undergoing differentiation and how it relates to the surrounding tissues will influence the result.

Fetal Growth Stage

This stage starts following the end of major organogenesis (day 45) and continues until term. The incidence of radiation-induced prenatal death and congenital aberrations during this stage is negligible. The main radiation-induced anomalies seen during this stage involve the nervous system and sense organs. This corresponds with their relative growth and development. Damage caused during this stage may not manifest itself until later in life, for example, behavioral changes, reduced IQ, or cancer.

Cancer Risk in Utero   In data obtained by Stewart in 1956 in a retrospective study of childhood cancer in Great Britain, referred to as the "Oxford survey of Childhood Cancers," a correlation was seen between childhood leukemia and solid tumors and irradiation in utero. Similar studies have confirmed this observation reporting a relative risk of approximately 1.4 for childhood cancer. This effect was not seen in the survivors of the atomic bomb who were irradiated in utero. These positive studies are widely disputed based on factors which include the influence of pre-existing medical conditions for which the exam was required and the lack of good estimates of fetal doses.

Human data have been examined by numerous national and international organizations who then developed risk estimates for carcinogenesis following in utero irradiation. **Neoplasm**s are estimated to be up to three times more frequent following irradiation in the first trimester as compared to the second and third trimesters. Peak occurrence of childhood leukemia was between the ages of 2–4 and was higher in males. An increased risk of childhood leukemia continued through the 10th year of life, compared to the 14th year for solid tumors, the majority of which were neoplasms of the

CNS. The current estimates for leukemia mortality are 2–3/10,000 after 1 rad (1 cGy) of low LET radiation. Solid tumors occur at approximately the same incidence. This brings the combined mortality from in utero irradiation to approximately 4–6/10,000 per rad (1 cGy). These mortality figures are thought to be identical to those cancers that occur spontaneously and in insufficient numbers to be easily identified in an exposed population.

In comparison, the natural total risk of mortality from malignancy through age 10 is 1/1200. If a fetus received a dose from a chest x-ray of 60 mrads (0.6 mGy), the chance of developing a fatal cancer during childhood from that exposure would be less than 1 in 27 million. The current effective dose equivalent limit to the fetus is no more than 500 mrem (5 mSv) during the gestational period, provided that the dose rate does not exceed 50 mrem (0.5 mSv) in any one month. If the maximum allowable dose was received, the chance of developing a fatal cancer during childhood from the exposure would be less than 1 in 3,300. While it is true that radiation exposure should be kept to a minimum, the risk at levels associated with occupational and diagnostic exposures is negligible when compared with other potential hazards.

Table 5–7 lists the effect of risk factors on pregnancy outcome.

Figure 5–6 depicts the relative incidence of radiation-induced health effects during the different stages of fetal development.

TABLE 5–7

EFFECT OF RISK FACTORS ON PREGNANCY OUTCOME[a]			
Effect	**Number Occurring from Natural Causes**	**Risk Factor**	**Excess Occurrences from Risk Factors**
	Radiation Risks		
	Childhood Cancer		
Cancer death in children	1.4/1,000	Radiation dose of 1,000 mrems received before birth	0.6/1,000
	Abnormalities		
		Radiation dose of 1,000 mrads received during specific periods after conception:	
Small head size	40/1,000	4–7 weeks > conception	5/1,000
Small head size	40/1,000	8–11 weeks > conception	9/1,000
Mental retardation	4,1,000	8–15 weeks > conception	4/1,000
			(continues)

TABLE 5-7 (continued)

EFFECT OF RISK FACTORS ON PREGNANCY OUTCOME[a]

Effect	Number Occurring from Natural Causes	Risk Factor	Excess Occurrences from Risk Factors
	Nonradiation Risks		
Occupation			
Stillbirth or spontaneous abortion	200/1,000	Work in high-risk occupation	90/1,000
	Alcohol Consumption		
Fetal alcohol syndrome	1–2/1,000	2–4 drinks/day	100/1,000
Fetal alcohol syndrome	1–2/1,000	More than 4 drinks/day	200/1,000
Fetal alcohol syndrome	1–2/1,000	Chronic alcoholic (>10 drinks/day)	350/1,000
Perinatal infant death	23/1,000	Chronic alcoholic (>10 drinks/day)	170/1,000
Smoking			
Perinatal infant death	23/1,000	Less than 1 pack/day	5/1,000
Perinatal infant death	23/1,000	One pack or more/day	10/1,000

[a]Source: U.S. Nuclear Regulatory Commission (NRC) Regulatory Guide 8.13, Rev. 2, *Instruction Concerning Prenatal Radiation Exposure*.

In utero irradiation risk can be put into perspective by examining the probability of birthing a healthy child after a given dose to the conceptus. Please refer to Table 5–8.

A fetal dose of even 1 rem (10 mSv) does not seriously affect the risks that are associated with pregnancy. Although therapeutic abortions because of fetal doses are rarely justified, each case should be analyzed individually and the risks explained to the patient. All efforts should be taken to reduce irradiation to the patient and especially the fetus. In looking at the relatively minute risk that is associated with diagnostic examinations, the postponement of clinically indicated examinations or scheduling examinations around the patient's menstrual cycle to avoid irradiation of a potential fetus are usually not warranted. Nevertheless, prior to diagnostic examinations that involve ionizing radiation, all fertile female patients should be questioned as to whether there is the possibility that they might be pregnant. If it is known that the patient is pregnant and alternative diagnostic procedures are not appropriate, the risks and benefits of the examination should be discussed with the patient prior to the examination.

FIGURE 5–6
Relative incidence of radiation-induced health effects during stages of fetal development (Adapted from Mettler, F. A., Moseley, R. D. *Medical effects of ionizing radiation*. New York: Grune & Stratton, 1985.)

TABLE 5–8

PROBABILITY OF HEALTHY CHILD AFTER GIVEN DOSE TO CONCEPTUS

Probability of Birthing Healthy Children[a]

Dose[b] to Conceptus (mSv [mrem])	Child with No Malformation (Percentage)	Child Will Not Develop Cancer (Percentage)	Child Will Not Develop Cancer or Have a Malformation (Percentage)
0 (0)	96	99.93	95.93
0.5 (50)	95.999	99.927	95.928
1.0 (100)	95.998	99.921	95.922
2.5 (250)	95.995	99.908	95.91
5.0 (500)	95.99	99.89	95.88
10.00 (1000)	95.98	99.84	95.83

[a]From Wagner L. K., Hayman L. A.: Pregnancy in women radiologists. *Radiology, 145*:599-562, 1982.
[b]Refers to absorbed dose above natural background. This table assumes conservative risk estimates, and it is possible that there is no added risk.

STOCHASTIC AND NONSTOCHASTIC EFFECTS

The biological effects of irradiation are classified as either **stochastic** or **nonstochastic** (deterministic). Stochastic effects occur randomly in nature. Also referred to as the statistical response, a stochastic effect is one where the probability of occurrence of effects, rather than their severity, increases with dose.

EXAMPLE

The chance of radiation-induced leukemia is considerably greater after an exposure to a dose at 100 rad (1 Gy) than at 1 rad (1 cGy), but there will be no difference in the severity of the disease if it occurs.

Stochastic effects are thought to be nonthreshold, as damage to a few cells or even a single cell could theoretically produce the disease. They are associated with the linear and linear quadratic dose-response curves. Therefore, even small exposures could carry some increased risk. Modern radiation protection programs are based on the assumption that risks are proportional to dose with no threshold. Stochastic effects are regarded as the main health risk from low-dose radiation from exposures in the diagnostic radiology department. Examples of stochastic effects include radiation-induced cancer and radiation-induced genetic effects.

If radiation exposure is high, the principal biological effects will be death of the cells caused by degenerative changes in the exposed tissue. If this is so, the severity of the injury, rather than its chance of occurring, increases with dose. These nonstochastic or deterministic effects are different from stochastic effects in that they need much higher doses to occur.

Nonstochastic or deterministic effects are thought to be threshold, as there are doses below which the effect is not observed. Examples of nonstochastic or deterministic effects from ionizing radiation are cataracts, erythema, fibrosis and hematopoietic damage. Nonstochastic effects are relevant to serious radiation accidents, but are not likely to occur from diagnostic imaging examinations or routine occupational exposure. Nonstochastic or deterministic effects increase in severity with dose, and thus are considered to be threshold.

KEY CONCEPTS

- The epidemiology of radiation exposure determines the incidence, distribution, and control of the disease in a particular population.
- Risk estimation models measure the amount of risk in a particular population at a particular point in time related to a particular disease.

- Cancer occurrences as a result of exposure to radiation are termed radiation-induced malignancies.
- Life span shortening is the result of chronic exposure to radiation that results in the premature death of an individual.
- Genetic damage as a result of radiation is determined through the study of mutations in chromosomes and genetic coding that resulted from exposure of unborn children to radiation while in utero.
- The fetus will suffer adverse effects of irradiation while in utero at various growth stages. Cells that are undergoing rapid development upon exposure will show increased abnormalities and susceptibility to radiation-induced malignancies later in life.
- Stochastic effects occur randomly; the probability of being affected increases with the dose. Nonstochastic effects are deterministic; the severity of the injury increases with the dose, not the chance of it occurring.

SECTION REVIEW

1. A whole body radiation dose given in a period of seconds to minutes produces a clinical pattern called
   a. mortality rate
   b. relative biological effectiveness
   c. acute radiation syndrome
   d. clinical body dose

2. When does the greatest radiation hazard to a fetus exist?
   a. first trimester
   b. second trimester
   c. third trimester

3. A reddening of the skin caused by radiation damage is referred to as
   a. epistaxis
   b. epilation
   c. erythema
   d. cataractogenesis

4. Which of the following is *not* an early response to irradiation?
   a. breast cancer
   b. skin erythema occurring 2 weeks postexposure
   c. intestinal distress occurring 1 week postexposure
   d. chromosome aberrations

5. The annual effective dose-equivalent limit for the fetus of an occupational worker is
   a. 0.001 rem
   b. 0.01 rem
   c. 0.5 rem
   d. 1.0 rem

CASE STUDY

An x-ray exam has been performed on a female who later determined she was pregnant at the time of x-ray exposure. Discuss the factors that affect her embryo's response to irradiation. Explain the possible principal effects of irradiation to her fetus.

A radiographer that is subjected to chronic low doses of radiation may be affected by its damaging effects if protection measures are not applied. The components and methods considered for minimizing patient exposure are also useful in reducing personnel exposure.

It is the responsibility of the radiographer to minimize ionizing radiation exposure to the patient. Even more essential is adoption of this responsibility into the everyday work habits and decision-making processes.

CHAPTER

6

Protection of Personnel

KEY TERMS

Agreement states

ALARA

Bone marrow dose

Controlled area

Cumulative timing device

Deadman type

Dose

Dosimetry

Early effect of radiation

Effective dose-equivalent limit

Entrance skin exposure (ESE)

Film badge

Gonadal dose

Intermittent fluoroscopy

Inverse square law

Ionization chamber

Joint Commission on the Accreditation of Healthcare Organizations (JCAHO)

Late effect of radiation

Lead equivalent

Personnel dosimeters

Pocket dosimeter

Primary protective barrier

Protective tube housing

Radiation protection

Scattered radiation

Secondary protective barriers

Skin dose

Thermoluminescent dosimeters (TLD)

Time of occupancy (T)

Uncontrolled area

Use (U)

Useful beam

Workload (W)

OBJECTIVES

Upon completion of this chapter, the reader should be able to:

- Discuss the rationale for radiation protection
- Explain personnel dosimeters, dosimetry reports, and duties of the radiation safety officer
- Define and calculate the dose-limiting recommendations for diagnostic radiology personnel
- Explain structural shielding construction and list the items that influence this construction
- Describe how to decrease the radiographer's exposure during a mobile radiographic examination
- Identify ways to lessen the radiographer's exposure during a fluoroscopic examination
- Discuss how using distance can decrease radiation exposure
- Illustrate the inverse square law
- Identify garments that can be worn to reduce radiation exposure and explain when such garments should be used
- List the people and methods that can help with patient immobilization during an x-ray exposure

RATIONALE FOR RADIATION PROTECTION

When humans are exposed to ionizing radiation, there is a risk of damage to our cells and our offspring. The purpose of radiation protection is to lessen the likelihood of such occurrences.

If human cells respond to a high **dose** of radiation within minutes, days, or weeks after exposure, this is termed an **early effect of radiation**. The primary early effects to humans include hematologic depression (decrease in number of blood cells), skin erythema (reddening of skin), epilation (hair loss), chromosome damage, (destruction of cell chromosomes), gonad dysfunction (impaired function of gonads), and death (irreversible cessation of vital bodily functions) (see Chapter 4). In modern diagnostic radiology, doses of this size are not experienced.

If damage to human cells is not detected for months or years after radiation exposure, this is termed a **late effect** of radiation. The primary late effects to humans include radiation-induced cancer and genetic effects (see Chapter 5). Exposure to intermittent low doses of radiation over a long period of time is what we experience in modern diagnostic radiology.

Effective absorbed dose-equivalent limits have been installed to reduce the possibility of the occurrence of early and late effects of radiation.

MONITORING OF PERSONNEL

Because radiology personnel have the potential to be exposed to ionizing radiation, they must be monitored to ensure that their levels of exposure remain well below the annual dose-equivalent limits. Monitoring of personnel is mandatory when personnel are likely to receive 10% of the annual effective dose-equivalent limit.

Measurement of ionizing radiation doses to personnel is termed **dosimetry. Personnel dosimeters** record external radiation doses. The three types of personnel dosimeters used in diagnostic radiology include **film badges, thermoluminescent dosimeters (TLD),** and **pocket dosimeters** (Figure 6–1). These devices are worn by radiology personnel during working hours. Film badges and TLDs are monitored monthly, and dosimetry reports are returned to the subscribing institution. This report documents the personnel's radiation dose equivalent for a specific month. The institution's (radiation safety officer) RSO reviews the monthly dosimetry report and posts it in an appropriate area. The RSO is responsible for seeing that personnel do not exceed occupational exposure limits.

Film Badges

Film badges are the most popular type of personnel dosimeter. They measure occupational radiation exposure. Film badges consist of a small piece of special radiation-dosimetry film, similar to dental film, contained in a light-proof packet. This film packet is enclosed inside a plastic holder, which can be clipped to a person's clothing. The film packet is changed monthly. Vari-

FIGURE 6–1
Film badge, thermoluminescent dosimeter ring, and collar badge (Courtesy of Tech/Ops Landauer, Inc.)

ous types of metal filters are placed inside the holder. These filters shield certain parts of the film that permit estimates of dosage and radiation energy. Shallow and deep doses can be calculated according to the amount of darkening of the film after processing.

Film badges must be worn at the collar level. If wearing a lead apron, the film badge must be worn at the collar level on the outside of the lead apron. This location is chosen because it is at the approximate level of the sternum, which receives the highest dose of radiation.

Film badges must be worn with the correct side of the badge facing forward. This allows the film badge company to determine whether the radiation dose received by the wearer came from the front or behind the wearer.

The company that supplies institutions with film badges provides a control badge, which is kept in a radiation-free area. It serves as a baseline when compared with the rest of the film badges after processing by the monitoring company. After processing, the monitoring company constructs a characteristic curve similar to those used to determine film speed and contrast.

When undergoing medical and/or dental radiographs as a patient, the film badge should never be worn. Badges should be stored away from sources of radiation, and must be kept away from excessive heat and high humidity. They must be worn only for the designated period of time, and only by the person assigned to that badge.

Film badges have been in use since the 1940s, are inexpensive, easily handled, easily processed, and provide a permanent record. They are only accurate at 10 mrem or above, and are susceptible to fog caused by temperature, light leaks, and humidity.

Thermoluminescent Dosimeters

Thermoluminescent dosimeters (TLD) contain lithium fluoride (LiF) or calcium fluoride (CaF_2) crystals. When exposed to ionizing radiation, these crystals store radiant energy when heated. As it is heated, the crystal releases energy as light, which is then measured by a machine that documents the radiation exposure based upon how much light is emitted. There is a direct relationship between the intensity of light emitted and the radiation dose received by the crystal.

TLDs are commonly worn as finger rings by nuclear medicine personnel to measure occupational exposure to their hands from handling radioisotopes.

TLDs are superior over film badges in that they:

- are nearly tissue equivalent
- can be worn for 3 months
- are reusable
- are extremely accurate
- are more sensitive than film badges, to approximately 5 mrem

The disadvantages of TLDs are that they are expensive, and once the crystals have been heated, they provide no permanent record.

Pocket Dosimeters

Pocket dosimeters are the most sensitive of the three types of personnel monitoring devices. They provide an instantaneous reading, but must be recalibrated daily. Also, they are only capable of a predetermined range. If exposure exceeds this range, any additional amounts of exposure cannot be documented.

Externally, a pocket dosimeter resembles a fountain pen. It has a pocket clip for attaching to the person's clothing (Figure 6–2). Inside the dosimeter is an **ionization chamber**. The chamber has a positive and a negative electrode. The electrodes and chamber are given a positive charge before use. There is a stationary electrode, and a moving electrode that is referred to as a hair or fiber. Giving a charge to the device with a charging base causes the fiber to be electrostatically repelled from a central electrode. This charge is calibrated until the fiber is set at zero on a visible scale. Ionization of air by radiation causes the hair to move. X- or gamma-radiation ionizes the air within the chamber, which neutralizes the charges present on the fiber and electrode. As the number of negative ions in the chamber increase, the charge on the hair reduces. This causes the hair to move closer to the stationary electrode. Pocket dosimeters are read by viewing a scale through an eyepiece located on the end of the dosimeter.

FIGURE 6–2

A pocket ionization chamber (Courtesy of Nuclear Associates division of Victoreen, Inc., Carle Place, NY)

Pocket dosimeters are normally used only in emergency situations in which an immediate reading is necessary. They may give false readings if subjected to trauma or high humidity.

Dosimetry Report

Film badges and TLDs are collected on a monthly basis, and personnel are supplied with new badges. The used badges are sent to the supplier for processing and exposure calculations.

Approximately one month after badges have been returned to the supplier, the RSO receives a film badge (dosimetry) report. These reports are posted in an area where they can be reviewed by personnel for review of their occupational exposures.

The following information is contained on the dosimetry report:

- personnel ID number
- monitor type (film badge vs. TLD)
- employee name and social security number
- birthdate and sex
- exposure period
- current exposure
- cumulative quarterly exposure
- cumulative annual exposure
- cumulative total exposure
- unused part of permissible accumulated dose

Dosimetry exposure figures are listed in millirems. An M on the dosimetry report means a minimal or possibly no exposure.

Should a monitored employee change employment, his employer must transfer the cumulative total exposures and the unused part of the permissible accumulated dose for this person to his new employer.

If the RSO determines an employee has received an overexposure based on the dosimetry report, the employee must be counseled by the RSO, and documentation placed in the employee's personnel file in case of the need for any future reference. The institution's radiation safety program should have a definition of the nature of an overexposure, as determined by the RSO. Guidelines for the facility's monitoring program are also established by the RSO. Any questions that arise about an institution's radiation safety program should be directed to the RSO. It is recommended that an institution's RSO be a qualified physicist. The RSO's duties include:

- receiving, using and disposal of radioactive material;
- conducting radiation surveys;
- monitoring personnel and areas;
- testing for leaking radiation;
- designing protective shielding;
- responses to radiation related emergencies;
- radioactive spill decontamination.

DOSE-LIMITING RECOMMENDATIONS

Shortly after the discovery of x-rays by Roentgen in 1895, people came to appreciate the contributions that x-rays would make in medicine. However, it was also soon demonstrated that there would be risks involved. The first fluoroscope users displayed elevated occurrences of skin cancer, cataracts, and lesions of the hands and fingers. In order to keep the risks in check, standards needed to be instituted.

In the early days of radiation use only short-term effects were acknowledged. Believing that there was a tolerance dose below which there would be no effects, the rationale was that doses should be restricted only in regards to the short term. The 1930s and 1940s saw standards for imaging being established. During this time period, an exposure of one roentgen (R)/day was permissible. Compared with today's exposure levels, this is approximately two times the amount a radiographer would acquire in one year.

With the possibility of long-term radiation risks being acknowledged, radiation protection policies are aimed at reducing the likelihood of short and long-term effects.   Present-day radiation protection guidelines are established on the philosophy of keeping exposures **as low as reasonably achievable (ALARA)**.

Various organizations are involved with radiation protection standards. Their contributions include scientific research reports on radiation and its effects, recommending standards, and making and enforcing guidelines at the state and federal levels. These organizations are identified in Table 6–1.

Based on recommendations made by these agencies, radiation exposure limits can be initiated by an act of Congress.

Currently, 29 states in the United States have agreements with the Nuclear Regulatory Commission (NRC) in taking the responsibility to enforce radiation protection guidelines through each state's respective department of health. These 29 states are known as **agreement states**. In nonagreement states, both the NRC and the state are responsible for enforcing radiation protection regulations.

All states, whether agreement or nonagreement states, have guidelines for the use of ionizing radiation equipment. Most states act according to regulations designed after the Suggested State Regulations for the Control of Radiation. The recommended regulations are made by the CRCPD, NRC, EPA, Department of Health and Human Services Public Health Service, and the FDA.

Federal government regulations allow diagnostic radiology personnel to receive an annual **effective dose-equivalent limit** of 5 rem (50 mSv) for whole-body occupational exposure. The public has an annual effective dose-equivalent limit of 0.5 rem (5 mSv). This amount is 1/10 the amount allowed for people exposed occupationally.

The reason for radiation workers being allowed a larger dose equivalent is that the radiology work force is a very small group when compared with the whole population. Hence, radiation workers may receive larger amounts of radiation than the general public acquires. Even though radiation work-

TABLE 6-1

RADIATION PROTECTION ORGANIZATIONS	
ORGANIZATION	DATE ESTABLISHED
International Labour Organization (ILO)	1919
International Commission on Radiological Units and Measurements (ICRU)	1925
International Commission on Radiological Protection (ICRP)	1928
National Council on Radiation Protection and Measurement (NCRP)	1929
United Nations Scientific Committee on Effects of Atomic Radiation (UNSCEAR)	1955
National Research Council Committee on the Biological Effects of Ionizing Radiation (BEIR)	1955
International Atomic Energy Agency (IAEA)	1957
Conference of Radiation Control Program Directors (CRCPD)	1968
U.S. Nuclear Regulatory Commission (NRC), originally established as the U.S. Atomic Energy Commission (AEC)	1940
U.S. Environmental Protection Agency (EPA)	1970
U.S. Food and Drug Administration (FDA)	1848
U.S. Occupational Safety and Health Administration (OSHA)	1971

ers may receive more radiation than the general public, the dose equivalent must be kept to a minimum whenever possible.

The effective dose-equivalent limit for a radiographer during any 13 week period is 3 rem (30 mSv). The annual effective dose-equivalent limit for the lens of the eye is 15 rem (150 mSv), and for all other organs is 50 rem (500 mSv).

Student radiographers under 18 years of age have an annual effective dose-equivalent limit of 0.1 rem (1 mSv).

The dose-limiting recommendations during pregnancy are: total effective dose-equivalent limit = 0.5 rem (5 mSv); effective dose-equivalent limit for 1 month = 0.05 rem (0.5 mSv).

If the mother would receive 500 mrem, the embryo or fetus would receive an equivalent of less than 10 mrem. Table 6–2 summarizes the dose limitations.

A pregnant employee must voluntarily in writing tell her employer that she is pregnant, and give the approximate conception date. This notification

TABLE 6–2

ANNUAL DOSE LIMITS	
OCCUPATIONAL EXPOSURES	**DOSE LIMITS**
Whole-body	5 rem (50 mSv)
Lens of eye	15 rem (150 mSv)
Skin/extremities	50 rem (500 mSv)
Whole-body cumulative (lifetime)	Age × 1 rem (Age × 10 mSv)
Fetus (nine-month)	0.5 rem (5 mSv)
Fetus (one-month)	0.05 rem (0.5 mSv)
Student < 18 years of age	0.1 rem (1 mSv)
PUBLIC EXPOSURE	
Infrequent exposure	0.5 rem (5 mSv)
Frequent exposure	0.1 rem (1 mSv)

allows her employer to try to limit the dose to the fetus during her pregnancy. A pregnant employee by no means should be removed from her duties. The employee's previous exposure history should be reviewed, her work environment analyzed to estimate the possibility of receiving exposures that would be greater than the 0.5 rem limit, and finally her work routines altered to lessen the likelihood of risks.

The cumulative whole-body effective dose-equivalent limit is calculated by multiplying one's age in years times 1 rem (10 mSv).

EXAMPLE

A radiation worker who is age 30 would be allowed a cumulative whole body dose equivalent of 30 rems. Age (30) × 1 rem = 30 rems.

These occupational exposures are made in keeping with the ALARA principle, that is, maintain radiation exposures as low as reasonably achievable. ALARA suggests the absolute absorbed dose-equivalent values are to be kept below the maximum amounts allowed. The most effective way for radiographers to do this is to use correct radiation protection procedures, that is, accurately placing and collimating the x-ray beam.

Radiographers should familiarize themselves with approximated doses of representative radiologic exams, as patients may inquire about how much exposure they are receiving.

Table 6–3 lists the representative quantities for various x-ray exams:

TABLE 6–3

EXPOSURE QUANTITIES FOR SPECIFIC X-RAY EXAMS

Exam	Skin Dose (mrad)	Mean Marrow Dose (mrad)	Gonad Dose (mrad)
PA Chest	10–20	2	<1
AP Abdomen	250–500	30	125
Skull	100–200	10	<1
Extremity	10–200	2	<1
Cervical Spine	150	10	<1
Lumbar Spine	300	60	225
Pelvis	150	20	150

The radiographer should know her department's protocol regarding the release of such information to patients. It may be that only the radiologist or RSO may release this information.

Patients may not necessarily want to know specifics on exposure, but instead may only want to be assured that whoever is performing their exam is knowledgeable regarding representative exposures for radiologic exams.

All facilities which receive accreditation by the **Joint Commission on Accreditation of Healthcare Organizations (JCAHO)** are required to monitor doses from diagnostic radiologic exams. It is also recommended by the Center for Devices and Radiological Health (CDRH) that diagnostic radiologic institutions be familiar with the amounts of radiation that are received by patients. Patient doses are usually reported in one of three methods. **Skin dose**, also referred to as **entrance skin exposure (ESE)**, is a measure of the radiation to a patient's skin at the entrance surface. Skin dose is the type of method most often used, because it is easy to measure. To get a skin dose measurement, a TLD is placed on the patient's skin in the center of the primary x-ray beam. Because of suspected genetic response to ionizing radiation, **gonadal dose** is vital. Measuring the dose to the gonads is also easy to measure. **Bone marrow dose** is critical as bone marrow is thought to be the target organ responsible for radiation-induced leukemia.

If the output intensity from the x-ray tube is known, patient dose can be determined. The output intensity of an x-ray tube varies directly with the mAs (milliampere second), directly with the square of the kVp (kilovolt peak), and inversely with the square of the distance from the focal spot.

$$\text{Output intensity} = \frac{K(mAs)kVp^2}{d^2}$$

The measurement of K, which is a constant, is recorded at 70 kVp and 40 inches.

Once K is determined,

$$\text{Output intensity (mR)} = K(\text{mR/mAs})(\text{mAs}_2) \frac{(\text{kVp}_2)^2}{(70)^2} \frac{(100 \text{ cm})^2}{(d_2)^2}$$

K = recorded value at 70 kVp and 40 inches

mAs_2 = new technique

kVp_2 = new technique

d_2 = new SID (source-image receptor distance)

EXAMPLE

The determined value for K is 10 mR/mAs at 70 kVp and 40 inches SID. For an extremity, 3 mAs and 55 kVp are used. What is the intensity?

$$(10 \text{ mR/mAs})(3 \text{ mAs}) \frac{(55)^2}{(70)^2} \frac{(40)^2}{(40)^2} = 10 \text{ mR} \times 3 \times 0.6 \times 1 = 30 \text{ mR}$$

The ESE (entrance skin exposure) for an x-ray projection can be approximated by using an ionization chamber. A digital dosimeter is exposed to the technique used for the specified projection. The formula for calculating an estimated ESE dose is:

$$\frac{\text{dosimeter exposure (mR)}}{\text{ESE (mR)}} = \frac{\text{SSD}^2}{\text{SDD}^2}$$

SSD = source to skin distance

SDD = source to detector distance

If a radiographer doubles the mAs, the radiation intensity doubles. Doubling the mAs also doubles the ESE (entrance skin exposure), as long as other factors are held constant.

The following is the formula for mAs and intensity:

$$\frac{\text{mAs}_1}{\text{mAs}_2} = \frac{I_1}{I_2}$$

EXAMPLE

If an original intensity was 200 mR, and mAs is increased from 10 to 20 mAs, what happens to the intensity? Doubling mAs should also double intensity.

$$\frac{10}{20} = \frac{200}{x} \qquad 10x = 4,000 \qquad x = 400 \text{ mR}$$

EXAMPLE

If an original intensity was 200 mR, and mAs is decreased from 100 mAs to 50 mAs, what happens to intensity? Decreasing mAs should also decrease intensity.

$$\frac{100}{50} = \frac{200}{x} \qquad 100x = 10,000 \qquad x = 100 \text{ mR}$$

Changing kVp affects radiation intensity by the square of the ratios of the kVps. The following is the formula for kVp and radiation intensity:

$$\frac{(kVp_1)^2}{(kVp_2)^2} = \frac{I_1}{I_2}$$

EXAMPLE

If 50 kVp produces an intensity of 200 mR, what will be the intensity at 100 kVp if no other factors are changed? Increasing kVp should also increase intensity.

$$\frac{(50)^2}{(100)^2} = \frac{200}{x} \qquad \frac{1}{4} = \frac{200}{x} \qquad x = 800 \text{ mR}$$

EXAMPLE

If 100 kVp produces an intensity of 800 mR, what will be the intensity at 70 kVp if no other factors are changed? Decreasing kVp should also decrease intensity.

$$\frac{(100)^2}{(70)^2} = \frac{800}{x} \qquad \frac{100}{49} = \frac{800}{x} \qquad 100x = 39,200 \qquad x = 392 \text{ mR}$$

PRINCIPLES OF PERSONNEL EXPOSURE REDUCTION

Reduction of an individual's exposure to ionizing radiation may be accomplished by application of three basic principles: (1) reduce the amount of **time** spent in the vicinity of the radiation source while it is operating, (2) increase the **distance** between the radiation source and the individual to be protected, and (3) interpose a **shielding** material, which will attenuate the radiation from the source. These three basic principles are sometimes referred to as the three cardinal rules of radiation protection.

Time

X-ray imaging equipment produces radiation only during the actual exposure used to form the image during a procedure. The time of exposure on a per-image basis is very short (typically much less than 1 second) during radiographic procedures. During fluoroscopic procedures, which are used when dynamic information is required, the x-ray source may be on (usually intermittently) for several minutes to as long as an hour or more. To minimize exposure to radiation, individuals should reduce the amount of time they spend in the vicinity of an operable radiation source. The simplest way to do this is to ascertain whether their presence is needed during the procedure. Whenever possible, individuals should remain behind protective barriers.

Distance

Increasing the distance between the individual and the source of radiation is an effective method to reduce exposure to radiation. As distance from the source of radiation is increased, the radiation level will decrease significantly. Maximizing the distance from an operable source of radiation is a particularly effective method of exposure reduction during mobile radiographic and fluoroscopic procedures.

Shielding

Shielding is used when neither time nor distance is effective in achieving the desired degree of reduction in exposure. By interposing any material between the source of radiation and the point at which it is desired to reduce the exposure, a certain reduction in exposure will be achieved. The degree of exposure reduction will depend on the physical characteristics of the material (atomic number, density, and thickness). For fixed x-ray imaging facilities the most common materials are lead and concrete. Such facilities are designed in accordance with specific recommendations (NCRP Report No. 49) depending on the configuration of the equipment, its intended use, and the surrounding area. Additional devices, such as mobile shields, lead-equivalent aprons and lead-equivalent gloves should be used when it is not possible to take advantage of fixed structural barriers.

STRUCTURAL SHIELDING CONSTRUCTION

The two types of fixed barriers are primary and secondary. **Primary protective barriers**, which are located perpendicular to the line of travel of the primary x-ray beam, in radiography up to 140 kVp, should consist of 1/16 inch lead (Pb) which extends up at least seven feet from the floor when the x-ray tube is five to seven feet from the wall.

Secondary protective barriers, which are located parallel to the line of travel of the primary x-ray beam, cover areas exposed only to scattered and leakage radiation, and require 1/32 inch lead (Pb) under the same operating conditions stated above. Plaster or concrete often serves as a secondary barrier without added lead.

Control booths are regarded as secondary barriers. X-rays have scattered at least two times before hitting the control booth, which causes a reduction of the x-ray beam to one-millionth of its original value.

The radiographer can observe the patient by looking through the lead glass window in the control booth. This leaded glass observation window should have the same lead equivalency as the adjacent wall. Lead glass is typically four times as thick as sheet lead for equivalent protection. Observation windows may be obtained in lead equivalencies from 0.3 to 2 mm. The average lead glass window of the shielded control booth consists of 1.5 mm Pb equivalent.

The exposure cord for the control booth must be short enough so that an exposure can be made only when the radiographer is entirely behind the control booth barrier. Control booth walls must be at least 7 feet high, and should be mounted permanently to the floor. If there is a door that is used as a necessary component of the control booth, it should be electrically interlocked with the control panel so that x-rays cannot be produced without the door being closed.

In addition to the primary and secondary protective barriers previously mentioned, the x-ray tube itself must be enclosed by a lead-lined metal covering, the required shielding being approximately 1.5 mm (1/16 inch) Pb. This **protective tube housing** serves to reduce leakage radiation to an assigned safe level. Leakage from the x-ray tube housing should not exceed 100 mR/hr at 3 feet (1 meter).

During radiography and fluoroscopic procedures, at 1 meter from the patient, the beam intensity is reduced by a factor of 1,000, to approximately 0.1% of the original beam intensity.

Factors which determine protective barrier thickness include distance, **time of occupancy (T), workload (W),** and **use (U).**

Barrier thickness depends on the distance between the radiation source and the barrier. This distance is that to the adjacent occupied area. The greater the distance between the radiation source and the barrier, the less thickness of lead the barrier.

Time of occupancy factor (T) denotes the amount of time a hospital area is occupied by people. Occupancy factor (T) is divided into two types: controlled and uncontrolled. A **controlled area** is an area occupied by radiation personnel. This area is always given an occupancy factor of 1. This is an implication that a radiation worker is always present. An **uncontrolled area** is one that is occupied by non-radiation personnel, that is, the general public. These areas are designated as either full, partial, or occasional, depending on their purpose. Stairways, unattended elevators, and outside areas are examples of uncontrolled areas.

The uncontrolled area occupancy factor value depends on the use of the area, for example, hallways = (T) factor of 1/4, stairways and unattended elevators = (T) factor of 1/16.

Controlled area design limits require barriers to reduce the exposure rate to less than 100 mrem/week. Uncontrolled area design limits require barriers to reduce the exposure rate to less than 10 mrem/week. Thus, uncontrolled walls must have approximately a tenth-value layer lead than a controlled wall.

Barrier thickness depends on the radiation level activity in that room. The more exams performed, the thicker the barrier needed. This characteristic, called workload (W), which takes into account weekly average tube current and tube operating time, is measured in milliampere-minutes/week (mA-min/wk). A small office may have workloads of less than 100 mA-min/wk, whereas a busy hospital may have a general purpose x-ray room with workloads as high as 500 mA-min/wk.

EXAMPLE

Plans for a private radiologist office call for two x-ray rooms. Patient load for each room is estimated to be 10 patients/day, with each patient averaging 4 films taken at 70 kVp, 70 mAs. What will be the projected workload of each room?

10 patients/day × 5 days/week = 50 patients/week
50 patients/wk × 4 films/patient = 200 films/week
200 films/week × 70 mAs/film = 14,000 mAs/week

$$14,000 \text{ mAs/week} \times \frac{1 \text{ minute}}{60 \text{ seconds}} = 233.3 \text{ mA-min/week}$$

The use factor (U) is the percentage of time which the x-ray beam is energized and directed toward a particular wall. The NCRP recommends that primary wall barriers be given a use factor of 1, and that primary floor barriers be given a use factor of 1. A wall that is not a primary barrier would be given a use factor of 1/4. Because scattered and leakage radiation are present 100% of the time when the x-ray tube is energized, the use factor for secondary barriers is assigned a factor of 1.

USE OF PROTECTIVE GARMENTS

Because lead's high atomic number assures that most scatter photons are absorbed, it is the material most often chosen for shielding.

Shields are evaluated by half- and tenth-value layers. HVLs and TVLs refer to the lead thicknesses that will reduce the intensity of radiation to 50% and 10%, respectively.

Lead aprons should be worn by all radiographers performing mobile and/or fluoroscopic procedures, and if holding a patient during an exposure. Aprons are composed of lead-impregnated vinyl or rubber. Lead aprons are manufactured in thicknesses of 0.25, 0.5, and 1 mm lead equivalencies. NCRP Report #102 maintains that lead aprons must be 0.5 mm Pb equivalent X-ray attenuation at 75 kVp for a 1 mm Pb equivalent apron is 99%.

Presuming the person wearing a lead apron is facing the primary x-ray beam, approximately 3/4 of the body's active bone marrow is covered. There are full wrap-around aprons available for personnel who are not always able to be facing the primary beam.

The greater the lead equivalency of an apron, the heavier it is for the person wearing it, which could possibly lead to back problems. 1 mm aprons may weigh up to 25 lbs.

To offset the weight factor of lead-impregnated aprons, manufacturers have begun to make aprons of composite materials. The aprons are made of a combination of barium, tungsten, and lead. This combination of materials maintains comparable radiation attenuation with lead aprons, and also is reduced in weight by almost 30%.

When wearing a lead apron, the personnel dosimeter should be worn at the collar level on the outside of the apron.

Maternity aprons are available for pregnant personnel. These aprons maintain 0.5 mm Pb equivalent protection throughout, and also contain an extra band of lead which covers the patient the entire width of the apron from the xiphoid process to slightly below the symphysis pubis. The additional band of lead provides the fetus with 1 mm Pb equivalent protection.

Pregnant radiographers should be provided with two personnel dosimeters. When wearing a lead apron, one should be worn at the collar level on the outside of the apron, and the other should be worn at the waist level on the inside of the apron.

If it is necessary for personnel to have their hands in the beam, lead gloves with a minimum lead equivalency of 0.25 mm must be worn. Sterile gloves which are radiation resistant are also manufactured. These are composed of lead-lined rubber. The thinness of the sterile glove permits more flexibility than is available with ordinary lead gloves, but they do not have the attenuation that regular lead gloves do.

Radiologists receive high radiation doses to the thyroid when performing fluoroscopy. Women tend to find a greater need to wear thyroid shields than men, as women are four times more likely to develop radiation-induced thyroid tumors. Thyroid shields of 0.5 mm lead equivalency are available to protect the thyroid area of personnel. Wearing a thyroid shield during fluoroscopy reduces the dose to the individual by a factor of 10.

Although protective eyewear has been recommended to be worn by radiologists during fluoroscopy to protect the eyes from cataractogenic effects of radiation, this need has never been established. Protective eyeglasses are available with lead equivalency protection of 0.35 mm.

MOBILE EXAM CONSIDERATIONS

It is crucial that the radiographer initiate effective communication with the patient during a mobile radiographic exam. Just as when performing an exam in the department, the radiographer should appraise the patient's condition and her capability to cooperate.

Before the radiographer makes an exposure during mobile radiography, she should instruct any people who are not required to be in the room during the exposure to leave the area. Anyone who is not able to leave the area during the exposure, including patients, must be provided with protective shielding. After the exposure is done, the radiographer should instruct anyone who was asked to leave the area that the exposure has been completed and that the room may be re-entered.

In order to receive the least amount of **scattered radiation** during a mobile exam, the radiographer should position herself at right angles to the scattering object (patient). Taking into consideration the radiation protection factors of distance and shielding, this is where the radiographer will receive the least amount of scattered radiation. The radiographer is also advised to take a position around a corner during the exposure. When doing so, any radiation that does reach the radiographer will have scattered at least two times. For each scattering effect, the radiation exposure is reduced by a factor of 0.01%. The radiographer would receive the greatest amount of radiation by standing beside the x-ray machine, because of backscatter exiting the patient.

Lead aprons should be worn at all times by radiographers performing mobile radiographic procedures. In accordance with NCRP Report #102, these lead aprons must have a minimum lead thickness of 0.5 mm. If the radiographers' hands have to be placed in the primary beam, lead gloves must be worn. These gloves must have a minimum lead thickness of 0.25 mm.

The mobile unit exposure switch must permit the radiographer to obtain a distance of at least six feet from the x-ray tube, patient, and useful beam. Utilizing distance takes advantage of the inverse square law. It is recommended that the radiographer stand at least six feet from the x-ray

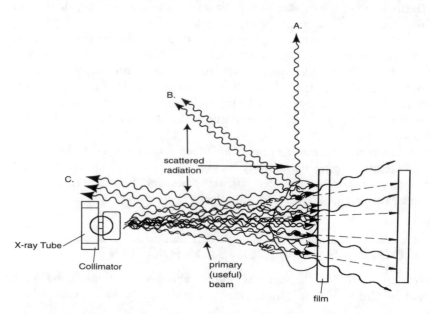

FIGURE 6–3

Sources of potential radiation during mobile exam

source. Sources of potential radiation during an exposure include both the x-ray tube and the patient Figure 6–3).

During mobile procedures, the radiographer should use a combination of the three cardinal principles of radiation protection: time, distance, and shielding.

- Reduce time: While the x-ray tube is operating, keep the amount of time spent in the area of the tube to a minimum.
- Increase distance: Keep as large a distance as possible between the energized x-ray tube and the exposed patient.
- Utilize shielding: Place lead shielding between the energized x-ray tube and the exposed person.

Table 6–4 summarizes some rules to remember when using mobile radiography.

FLUOROSCOPIC EXAM CONSIDERATIONS

A lead apron of at least 0.25 mm Pb equivalent must worn by all persons (other than the patient) who are present in the fluoroscopic room during

TABLE 6-4

RADIATION PROTECTION RULES FOR MOBILE RADIOGRAPHY

1. Recognize a duty to protect your patient, health professionals, physicians, the public and yourself.

2. Request the public, health professionals, physicians and other patients to leave the immediate area prior to exposure.

   (Always inform these persons that you will be finished in a moment, request them to remain nearby, and inform them promptly when you are finished.)

3. Announce in a loud voice your intent to make each exposure and permit sufficient time for others to leave.

4. Carry at least two lead aprons: one for yourself, the other for your patient. If you have an assistant, he too must have an apron.

5. Never place your hand or any other body part within the primary beam.

6. Provide gonadal protection for your patient.

7. Achieve maximum distance from the patient (not the tube) immediately prior to exposure, in accordance with rules requiring the use of a 6' cord on mobile units.

8. Label and handle each cassette carefully to avoid repeats.

(From Carlton, R. & Adler, A. [2001]. *Principles of radiographic imaging: An art and science* (3rd ed.). Albany, NY: Delmar Thomson Learning.)

exposure. An apron designed to cover the front and sides of the body is usually sufficient, although a wrap-around apron for both front and back should be considered if the radiographer is required to turn his/her back to the patient and x-ray tube during the procedure. Radiographers assisting during fluoroscopy must develop the ability to back and sidle around the room during exposures, always keeping the front of the body with its lead apron facing the patient and tube. If the hands must be placed within the primary beam, lead gloves of at least 0.25 mm Pb equivalent must be worn.

The primary source of exposure to the radiographer and radiologist is the patient. It is worth noting that the highest energy scatter occurs at a 90° angle to the incident beam and that the patient on an x-ray table is usually at the same level (90° from a primary photon angle of incidence) as the gonads of the radiographer. It is also worth remembering that according to the inverse square law, a single step back from the patient will decrease the dose exponentially. The slot immediately under the tabletop where the Bucky tray is positioned for diagnostic radiography is also at the gonadal level. Fluoroscopic units must have a lead shield to cover this slot. However, it must be brought into position by moving the Bucky tray to the head or foot of the table prior to beginning fluoroscopy. Strips of lead rubber, forming a drape are positioned between the fluoroscopist and patient to absorb the majority of the patient scatter. The radiographer has one advantage during fluoroscopy in that he/she may position himself/herself behind the radiologist. This not only adds an additional lead apron, but the entire body of the fluoroscopist is there to protect the radiographer.

Fluoroscopy units with cassette spot filming devices are available in front and rear loading models. The front loading models require the fluoroscopist to eject the cassette and lift the arm to permit the radiographer to remove the exposed cassette and insert an unexposed replacement. During this procedure it is difficult to operate the fluoroscopic unit, but if it is operated the radiographer is protected from scatter by a lead drape, the fluoroscopist, and the fluoroscopist's lead apron as well as his/her own lead apron. Rear loading models require the radiographer to lift the exposed cassette from the rear of the carriage. This usually requires stepping onto a platform at the rear of the fluoroscopy table and places the radiographer within inches of the patient (the source of scatter radiation). Fluoroscopy units should not be operated during replacement of spot film cassettes from rear loading units.

The fluoroscopic exposure switch is controlled by the radiologist by using either a foot pedal, or a hand switch located on the fluoro carriage. The switch is considered a **deadman type**. Only when constant pressure is applied by the radiologist will the fluoroscope tube emit radiation.

The source-to-tabletop distance must not be less than 30 cm (12 inches) for mobile fluoroscopic units, and not less than 38 cm (15 inches) for fixed fluoroscopic units.

The total filtration of the fluoroscopic equipment must be at least 2.5 mm Al equivalent.

The image intensifier component acts as a primary protective barrier and should be at least 2 mm **lead equivalent** (Pb eq).

A **cumulative timing device** must be provided that produces an audible signal when five minutes of fluoroscopic time have been used. This timer is reset with each five minutes of use, and also with each new fluoro procedure.

The fluoroscopic x-ray intensity at the tabletop must not exceed 10 R/min.

The radiologist is trained to use **intermittent fluoroscopy**, and also should collimate so as to include only the area of interest. This is done to reduce the radiation exposure to the patient.

The best way of reducing radiation exposure to personnel during fluoroscopy is distance. When the radiographer is assigned to fluoroscopy, he/she should step back from the fluoroscopic table whenever not immediately needed and assistance is not required. The use of high kVp is the second choice of reducing exposure to personnel during fluoroscopy.

INVERSE SQUARE LAW

By increasing the distance between the radiation source and the radiographer, the radiation exposure is decreased dramatically. This exposure decrease is calculated by using the **inverse square law**. This law states that the intensity of radiation at a given distance from a point source is inversely proportional to the square of the distance of the object from the source.

The inverse square law is represented mathematically as:

$$\frac{I_1}{I_2} = \frac{d_2^{\,2}}{d_1^{\,2}}$$

where I_1 = original distance exposure intensity

I_2 = new distance exposure intensity

d_1 = original distance from source

d_2 = new distance from source

EXAMPLE

When the distance from the x-ray target is doubled, the radiation at this new distance covers an area four times as large as the original area. The x-ray exposure (intensity) at this new distance is 1/4 as much as the original exposure (intensity). This is demonstrated in Figure 6–4.

The bottom surface, represented by ABCD, is 2X the distance from the radiation source, and covers an area 4X the surface area of the upper surface, represented by abcd.

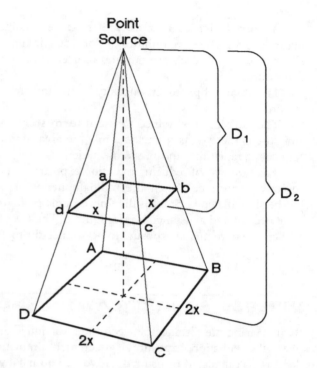

FIGURE 6–4
The inverse square law states that the intensity of radiation at a given distance from a point source is inversely proportional to the square of the distance. The lower surface area (ABCD) is twice as far from the source of radiation and is four times (2^2) the surface area of the upper surface area (abcd).

EXAMPLE

If a radiographer stands 2 feet from an x-ray tube, and receives an exposure of 1 mR/hr, what will be the exposure if the radiographer stands 4 feet from the x-ray tube?

$$\frac{I_1}{I_2} = \frac{d_2^2}{d_1^2}$$

$$\frac{1}{x} = \frac{4^2}{2^2}$$

$$\frac{1}{x} = \frac{16}{4}$$

Cross multiply the fractions.

$$16x = 4$$

To solve for x, divide each side by 16.

$$\frac{16x}{16} = \frac{4}{16}$$

$$x = \frac{1}{4}$$

Whenever possible, the radiographer should utilize the inverse square law, by increasing his/her distance from the exposure source, to reduce exposure from the source of radiation.

Also suggested by the inverse square law is that if a radiographer moves closer to a radiation source, the radiographer's radiation exposure will increase significantly.

EXAMPLE

If the radiographer positions himself 3 feet from the radiation source instead of 6 feet from the source, the radiation exposure to the radiographer increases by a factor of 4, according to the principles of the inverse square law.

Of the three cardinal principles of radiation protection, the inverse square law is the most effective means of protecting the radiographer from radiation exposure.

PATIENT IMMOBILIZATION CONSIDERATIONS

Immobilization of the patient may be necessary if there is voluntary motion. Involuntary motion is dealt with by using a short exposure time with a high mA selection.

A combination of proper communication and the use of positioning aids should be utilized. These aids include tape, angle sponges, sandbags, and foam pads. Sheets, towels, stockinettes, compression bands, and tape may be used on pediatric patients.

Immobilization must be used on patients who are not able to cooperate. The radiographer should determine the extent of the patient's ability to cooperate. A proper method of immobilization is then decided upon by the radiographer.

As a last resort, humans may be utilized to immobilize patients. Radiographers should be the last preference for patient immobilization. No one person should routinely hold patients.

The first choice for holding a patient is a friend or relative, preferably a male, since a male cannot be pregnant. Nonradiology hospital employees are the next choice. The final choice for holding patients would be radiology personnel.

Persons holding a patient for an exposure must be furnished with a lead apron, lead gloves, and a monitoring device. If a monitoring device is not available, there must be documentation of the procedure performed and the exposure factors used. The person holding the patient should be instructed to not stand in the useful/primary beam during the exposure. It is recommended by the ICRP that the person holding the patient be above the reproductive age. Under no circumstances should a pregnant female be used to support or hold a patient during an exposure.

In actuality, because of time constraints and lack of nonoccupational persons available to provide patient restraint, radiographers are utilized to restrain patients. Although this is a last resort, radiographers do expedite the exam by knowing exactly how to position the patients while at the same time restraining them, and also by communicating with the radiographer who is positioned at the control panel as to when to make the exposure. If this is the case, the radiographer who is restraining the patient must wear a lead apron, lead gloves, and a radiation monitor located at the collar level outside of the lead apron, and should position himself so as to not stand in the primary beam. This holding of the patient must be documented.

Many medical facilities keep a daily logbook in which is recorded the patient's name, date exam was performed, exposure technique factors, number of films taken, and radiographer's initials. Also recorded is the name of human immobilizer used, and during which exposures they were utilized.

If physical restraint is to be used on a patient, you must first get his/her consent. Failing to do so may result in legal consequences.

Permitting patients to cooperate if they are able to do so is recommended. Achieving patient cooperation and consent may save you from having to do repeat films. All radiographers should employ this professional approach when giving patient instructions.

KEY CONCEPTS

- Radiation protection is used to limit the amount of radiation an individual is exposed to, thus warding off ill effects of the radiation exposure.
- Personnel dosimeters are devices worn by radiographers to measure the amount of radiation they are exposed to on a daily basis. Dosimeter reports summarize the amount of radiation an individual is exposed to in a specific period. The radiation safety officer is responsible for maintaining the protection of personnel, monitoring personnel exposures, testing for radiation leaks, developing shielding apparatus, responding to emergencies involving radiation exposure, and decontamination of radiation spills.
- Dose-limiting recommendations were developed to ensure that personnel are only exposed to the minimum levels to maintain health. This is calculated by multiplying one's age in years by 1 rem.
- Structural shielding construction develops an area to provide the maximum amount of safety for the radiographer by limiting the exposure of radiation by use of barriers. Factors to consider when developing these areas are distance, time of occupancy, workload, and use.

- To reduce the amount of exposure of the radiographer during a mobile exam, the radiographer should wear a lead apron, be at least six feet away from the patient, and position himself at right angles to the patient. It is also advisable to take a position around a corner from the patient.
- To minimize exposure of the radiographer during a flouroscopic exam, the radiographer should try to increase the distance from the table.
- Increasing one's distance decreases exposure as a result of the radiation scattering.
- The inverse square law is used to measure the decease in exposure by increasing distance. The intensity of radiation at a given distance is inversely proportional to the square of the distance of the object from the source.
- Lead aprons, lead gloves, thyroid shields, and protective eyewear should be worn to protect against exposure to radiation.
- When a patient needs to be immobilized, individuals who are not regularly exposed to radiation should be used first. Radiographic personnel should be used only as a last resort. Positioning aids can also be used such as tape, sponges, sandbags, and foam pads.

Protection of Patients

OBJECTIVES

Upon completion of this chapter, the reader should be able to:

- Discuss the importance of immobilization of the patient during an x-ray exposure
- Describe beam-limiting apparatus and name the mechanism which best limits the x-ray beam
- Explain the purpose of x-ray beam filtration in diagnostic radiography
- State the reasons for using gonadal shielding during radiologic examinations and recognize the varieties of shields employed
- Discuss the necessity for using correct exposure factors for all radiologic procedures
- Demonstrate how the use of high speed film-screen combinations decreases radiographic exposure to the patient
- Explain the rationale for decreasing the number of repeat radiographs
- Discuss how patient exposure may be reduced during fluoroscopic procedures

IMMOBILIZATION

If there is patient movement during an x-ray exposure, there will be blurring of the radiographic image, and the radiologist will be unable to obtain an accurate diagnosis from such a film. The consequence of this would be a repeat exposure, resulting in twice the radiation to the patient and radiographer.

The need for repeat exposures can sometimes be the result of lack of communication between the patient and radiographer. The patient should be advised that a procedure may cause discomfort or possibly unusual feelings. A communication gap may occur as the result of insufficient or poorly interpreted instructions. Competent directions between the radiographer and the patient can help to prevent the need for repeat radiographs.

An example of this might be a barium enema exam. The radiographer should explain to the patient that there might be some minimal discomfort as the barium sulfate is administered into the colon, but that any discomfort will soon subside. The patient should be instructed that to avoid any possible repeat x-rays, it is necessary to try to control any **voluntary motion** during the study while experiencing any discomfort.

To reduce voluntary patient motion, the radiographer should use immobilization techniques during the radiation exposure. There are numerous products which are available for this purpose. These immobilization devices may be necessary when radiographing infants (Figure 7–1), and when examining patients who are incapacitated and thus unable to cooperate with the radiographer in not moving during the exposures

When dealing with **involuntary** patient **motion**, the radiographer should reduce radiation exposure times along with using immobilization mechanisms.

FIGURE 7–1
Pediatric immobilization devices

If the part being studied moves during the x-ray exposure, the result is motion unsharpness. Motion unsharpness can be restricted by using as short an exposure time possible.

Examples of involuntary patient motion would be heart contraction/relaxation, and bowel peristalsis. The best way to reduce the chance of such involuntary patient motion is the use of minimal exposure times.

BEAM RESTRICTION

Scatter radiation is produced during a Compton interaction. In this interaction, a primary photon interacts with an outer-shell electron and changes direction, thereby becoming a scattered photon. Proper beam restriction will keep the total amount of tissue irradiation to a minimum and has great importance in both improving image quality and reducing patient dose.

As the beam is restricted, fewer primary photons are emitted from the tube and collimator and fewer scattered photons are created. Additionally, the decrease in the number of primary photons results in a decrease in the dose to the patient.

The principal factors that affect the amount of scatter produced are 1) kilovoltage and 2) the irradiated material. In order to control the amount of scatter produced, it is important to understand how kilovoltage and the irradiated material affect scatter production.

Kilovoltage

Kilovoltage affects the penetrability of the beam. As kVp increases, fewer photons undergo interaction with matter and more pass through the patient to interact with the film. For the photons that undergo an interaction, the photoelectric absorption and Compton interactions are predominant in the diagnostic x-ray range. Although the total number of photons that undergo interaction decreases with increased kVp, a shift is seen in the percentage of photoelectric versus Compton interactions as kVp increases. As the kilovoltage increases, the percentage of x-rays that undergo a Compton interaction increases and the percentage of photons that undergo photoelectric absorption decreases. Because Compton interactions create scatter, as kilovoltage increases the percentage of primary photons that will undergo scattering also increases. At the same time, the percentage of primary photons that are absorbed photoelectrically decreases, resulting in a reduction in patient dose.

In radiography, the kilovoltage level is selected based predominantly on the size of the part being examined and the radiographic contrast desired for the image. When kilovoltage is increased without any other changes in technical factors, more scatter will result. If, however, the increase in kilovoltage is accompanied by a reduction in mAs to maintain the same dose, the overall result will be a decrease in the amount of scatter produced. Overall fewer photons are needed to create an acceptable image.

Irradiated Material

The amount of scatter created during an interaction is affected by the volume and atomic number of the material being irradiated. The volume of irradiated material is controlled by field size and patient thickness.

As the volume of irradiated tissue increases, the amount of scatter increases. Volume increases as the field size increases or as the patient thickness increases. Larger field sizes, such as with 14" × 17" (35 × 32 cm) film, allow for more photons to interact with tissue, thereby creating more scatter. Larger body parts have more tissue to interact with the photons, resulting in greater scatter production. In order to decrease scatter, the smallest possible field size should be used. It is for this reason that beam restriction is an important part of scatter reduction and, of course, patient protection.

BEAM-LIMITING DEVICES

Decreasing the area of the x-ray beam helps to reduce absorbed and scattered radiation by the patient. This is accomplished by using x-ray beam limiting apparatus called diaphragms, **cones**, and collimators.

Aperture Diaphragms

The simplest type of **beam limitation device** is the **aperture diaphragm**. It is a piece of flat lead containing a hole in its center. Attached to the tube head, it confines the x-ray beam so that a 1 cm unexposed border is visible on all sides of the finished radiograph (Figure 7–2). Aperture diaphragms are used in special procedure angiography studies.

FIGURE 7–2

Aperture diaphragm

Cones

Cones are circular metal structures that attach to the x-ray tube housing to restrict the x-ray beam to a predetermined circular size. They may be either a straight tube or a flared cylinder (Figure 7–3 A & B). Cones are used for lateral sella turcica films, sinuses, L5/S-1 spine radiographs, and dental radiography. The greatest beam limitation occurs with the longest cone and smallest diameter available. Metal and/or lead cones may also be used in dental radiography. The use of lead-lined cones results in the least exposure to the patient.

Collimators

The most broadly used beam restricting device is the **variable-aperture collimator**. They are composed of an upper and lower pair of lead shutters. The shutters are at right angles to each other and move independently of the other pair (Figure 7–4). They may be adjusted to numerous square or rectangular field sizes. Variable shutter type collimators also contain a lamp and a mirror. The lamp provides a light source to illuminate the area of interest, and the mirror is used to deflect the light toward the patient

FIGURE 7–3 A

Cones

FIGURE 7–3 B
Cones

First stage
entance shutters

Rotating anode

Fixed barrier

Focal spot

Outline of
collimator
housing

Port of x-ray tube housing

Mirror

Mirror first stage
long shutters

Second stage
cross shutters

Image
receptor

Useful beam

Extrafocal
radiation

FIGURE 7–4
Reducing light field to area of clinical
interest

anatomy. A cross-hair in the light field marks the center of the x-ray beam. Collimators are the most widely used beam restricting device because they contain a light source which helps the radiographer to correctly center the x-ray beam on the specific area to be radiographed. They also regulate the field size to the anatomical structure of interest. The purpose of the lead shutters is to restrict x-ray field size. The upper shutters absorb off-focus radiation before it leaves the x-ray tube. The lower shutters are mounted below the lamp and mirror, and further restrict the x-ray beam to the area of interest. Reducing the light field to only the area of clinical interest helps to reduce unnecessary patient exposure.

Equipment may be supplied with automatic collimation devices that are electronically interlocked with the Bucky tray so that the x-ray beam size is automatically restricted to the cassette size in use (Figure 7–5). Accuracy within 2% of the SID is required with automatic collimation devices (2% × 100 cm = 0.02 × 100 = 2 cm). When correctly adjusted, automatic collimation causes an unexposed border on all sides of the radiograph.

X-RAY BEAM FILTRATION

In conventional x-ray tubes, to assist in reducing patient exposure, an aluminum filter is inserted in the path of the x-ray beam. Filters absorb low energy photons, which improves the beam quality and increases average beam energy (hardness).

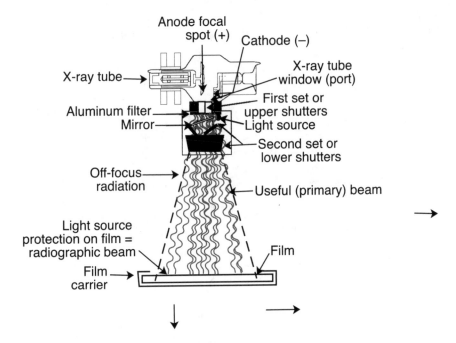

FIGURE 7–5
Unexposed border on all sides of radiograph

Since filtration absorbs some x-ray photons, it decreases the intensity of radiation. The photons not absorbed by the filtration are more penetrating and have less chance of being absorbed by the body. Thus, the patient absorbed dose is decreased when correct filtration is placed in the x-ray beam path. If proper filtration is not used, low energy x-ray photons are absorbed by the body (Figure 7–6).

The two types of filtration are inherent and added. **Inherent filtration** consists of the glass window of the x-ray tube and the cooling oil surrounding the tube housing. **Added filtration** consists of aluminum or aluminum equivalent (Al eq.) of appropriate thickness inserted outside the glass window of the tube housing. The combination of inherent filtration plus added filtration equals **total filtration**. Inherent filtration increases as the tube ages.

The peak kilovoltage of an x-ray unit is the determining factor for the total filtration required (Figure 7–7).

Requirements for filtration in fixed radiographic equipment are:

Operating kVp	Minimum Total Filtration in mm Al eq.
Below 50	0.5
50-70	1.5
Above 70	2.5

The minimum total filtration for mobile diagnostic and/or fluoroscopic units is 2.5 mm Al eq.

To verify whether a diagnostic x-ray beam is adequately filtered, the **half-value layer (HVL)** of the beam must be measured. The HVL is the thickness of material which will reduce the x-ray intensity to half its original value. This measurement is obtained by quality control personnel on an

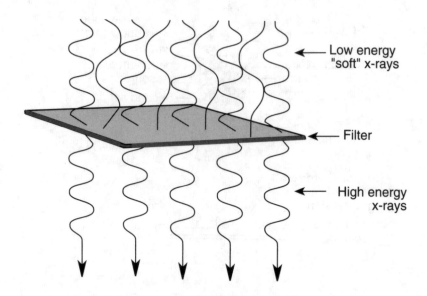

← Low energy "soft" x-rays

← Filter

← High energy x-rays

FIGURE 7–6

Filtration absorbing low energy photons

FIGURE 7–7

Filtration requirements for kVp levels

annual basis, and also after repairs have been performed on the tube housing or collimator systems. The HVL is a characteristic of the x-ray beam and measures the beam quality.

An example of this would be to assume an original tube intensity of 100 mR. If one HVL is added, the new intensity would be 50 mR, or equal to one-half the original intensity.

Table 7–1 shows the change in HVL with increase in kVp for fixed radiographic units having 2.5 mm Al total filtration.

GONADAL SHIELDING

The first step in providing gonad protection for a patient during an x-ray exposure is to properly collimate the x-ray beam to include only the area of clinical interest. Gonad shields should be used when the gonads are in or within 5 cm of the primary x-ray beam. **Gonad shielding** should be utilized for anyone thought to be within the reproductive age. The breasts, gonads, and lens of the eye are often shielded from the primary x-ray beam.

TABLE 7–1

CHANGE IN HVL WITH INCREASE KVP	
kVp	HVL (mm Al)
50	1.9
75	2.8
100	3.7
125	4.6

Gonadal shielding should not be used when it interferes with necessary diagnostic information.

The types of gonadal shields are flat, contact, shadow, and shaped contact (Figure 7–8).

Flat Contact Shields

Flat contact shields are composed of rubberized lead strips. These are laid directly over the patient's gonads, and may be secured to the patient with tape if necessary. These shields are useful for simple recumbent studies.

Shadow Shields

Shadow shields consist of a radiopaque material. This type of gonad shield is suspended from the x-ray tube housing, casting a shadow over the gonadal area. These shields are useful when encountering sterile fields, such as in the operating room.

Shaped Contact Shields

Shaped contact shields consist of lead. These are worn by male patients, and are held in place by some type of disposable supporter. The shield is placed into a pouch inside the supporter. These shields are useful when doing oblique, lateral, and erect studies. They may be used during fluoroscopic stomach studies. It is rare to find these currently in use.

EXPOSURE AND TECHNIQUE FACTORS

The radiographer can significantly reduce the approximate entrance skin exposure to the patient by judicious selection of technique exposure factors. Studies have shown that over 50% of repeated exposures are the result of improper technical factor selection. Table 7–2 illustrates the effect each

FIGURE 7–8
Gonadal shields: (left to right) flat shield, shadow shield, and shaped contact shield.

of the major technical factors has on patient dose. In most instances when a technical factor is varied, other factors will be modified to maintain

TABLE 7-2

EFFECTS OF RADIOGRAPHIC EXPOSURE VARIABLES ON PATIENT DOSE

		Effect of Patient Dose When:	
		Variable Is Increased but Radiograhic Density Is Maintained by Compensating	
Variable	Variable Is Increased Without Compensation	with kVp Only	with mAs Only
Kilovoltage	+	NA	–
Milliamperage	+	+	0
Time	+	+	0
Distance			
SID	–	–	0
SOD	–	–	0
OID	+	+	+
Focal spot size	0	NA	NA
Filtration	–	–	+
Field Size	+	varies	varies
Gonadal shielding	–	NA	NA
Subject part density	+	+	+
Grid Ratio	0	+	+
Intensifying screens	0	–	–
Film speed	0	–	–
Film processing			
Developer time	0	–	–
Developer temperature	0	–	–
Developer replenishment	0	–	–

(From Carlton, R. & Adler, A. [2001]. *Principles of radiographic imaging: An art and science.* Albany, NY: Delmar Thomson Learning.)

radiographic density. Therefore, the important information is not the direct result of the technical factor change, but the result of compensation to maintain radiographic density or other components of image quality.

Kilovoltage Range

When kVp is increased without compensating for other factors, patient dose is increased. Therefore, a decrease in kVp is desired when attempting to reduce patient dose. However, when an increase in kVp is compensated for by a decrease in mAs to maintain radiographic density, a significant reduction in patient dose is achieved. Selection of the highest possible kilovoltage consistent with image quality is the best method of using exposure factors to reduce patient dose. With fixed kilovoltage systems, care must be taken to achieve an optimal kVp that is within acceptance limits. Because fixed kVp technique systems tend to utilize higher optimal kVp levels, they usually reduce patient entrance skin exposures.

Remember that generator phase also has an effect on kilovoltage output. Although an increase in the number of pulses from the generator would seem to increase the patient dose because of the increased average photon energy, there is actually a substantial decrease in patient ESE (from 40 to 6%) because of the decrease in the percentage of lower energy photons from the x-ray tube. The lower energy photons tend to be absorbed in the body instead of being transmitted to the image receptor, thus contributing to patient ESE without adding any information to the image receptor.

Milliamperage and Time

When mAs is decreased, patient dose is also decreased. When an increase in mAs is compensated by a decrease in kVp, patient dose will increase. An inverse relationship exists between mAs and kVp in maintaining radiographic density. To decrease patient dose, mAs should be maintained at the lowest possible level because there is a direct relationship between mAs and exposure. Because variable kVp technique systems tend to utilize lower kVp levels with higher mAs, the result can be higher average patient ESE than with fixed kVp systems.

The use of high kVp and low mAs will result in reducing the absorbed dose to the patient (Figure 7–9). The technique selected should provide adequate part penetration, acceptable film density, and proper radiographic contrast.

FILM-SCREEN CONSIDERATIONS

A significant reduction in patient exposure results from using the highest speed **intensifying screens** and films consistent with satisfactory image quality. An example of this would be use of high speed intensifying screens and films during GI studies.

A.

High kVp, low mAs

X-ray tube

← High energy, penetrating x-ray beam

B.

Low kVp, high mAs

X-ray tube

← Low energy x-ray beam

FIGURE 7–9
Use of high kVp and low mAs to reduce absorbed dose

EXAMPLE

A lateral skull x-ray is taken at 65 kVp and 50 mAs, which results in a skin dose of 300 mrad. If the kVp is increased to 75 (a 15% increase), and the mAs is reduced by 1/2, to 25 mAs, the radiographic density should remain the same. (This technique adjustment would cause an increase in exposure latitude, and a decrease in contrast.) What is the patient skin dose? Answer:

Dose = (300 mrad)(25mAs/50mAs)(75kVp/65kVp) = (300 mrad)(0.5)(1.33) = 200 mrad.). (Caution should be taken when kVp is decreased and mAs increased, as there may not be adequate penetration using the new lower kVp).

Radiographic Film

Film is constructed at different speeds for use with intensifying screens that enhance the action of x-rays. Film speed influences radiographic exposure time. Increasing film speed means less exposure is required to obtain an image. With this decrease in exposure, there is a decrease in patient dose.

Intensifying Screens

Intensifying screens accelerate the action of x-rays by converting x-ray energy into visible light. Because a single x-ray photon can produce 80–95 light photons from an intensifying screen, this conversion speeds up the film exposure process. Approximately 95% of the density of a recorded image results from the visible light photons emitted by the intensifying screens. Because more light is emitted from the screens, radiographic exposure can be reduced. This leads to a reduction in patient dose.

Rare-earth intensifying screens are more efficient than calcium tungstate intensifying screens in converting x-ray energy photons into light photons. The rare-earth screens absorb three to five times more x-ray energy than calcium tungstate screens, thereby emitting more light. Rare-earth screens are from two to ten times faster than calcium tungstate screens. This increase in speed significantly reduces patient dose. Rare-earth screens are widely used in GI radiography.

Kilovoltage affects screen speed. As kVp increases, screen speed increases. This results in a reduction in patient dose.

PATIENT POSITIONING

An effective method of reducing patient dose is through accurate and effective positioning. Avoidance of repeated exposures far outweighs all other methods. However, once positioning skills have been developed to a degree of competence, several positioning details may further reduce the total dose.

Some organs are especially sensitive to the effects of radiation, for example, the female breast, the kidneys and the lens of the eye. Increased recorded detail and decreased distortion result when the area of interest is placed as close to the image receptor as possible. In most instances a significant reduction in the total dose is achieved because this positioning also places the organ as far from the entrance exposure as possible.

GRIDS

Radiographic grids are placed between the patient and the image receptor to preferentially absorb scatter radiation. Because grids absorb primary as well as scatter radiation, technical factors must be increased to produce an image of acceptable film density. This increase in technical factors results in an increase in patient dose but image quality is significantly improved. The lowest possible grid ratio consistent with effective scatter removal should be utilized to keep patient dose as low as reasonably achievable.

THE PREGNANT PATIENT

To minimize the possible exposure to an embryo in the earliest days of a pregnancy, a guideline known as the ten-day rule was recommended by a number of advisory agencies. This guideline stated that elective abdominal x-ray examinations of fertile women should be postponed until the ten-day period following the onset of menstruation as it would be improbable that a woman would be pregnant during these days. Based on the current understanding of radiobiology, this rule is now considered obsolete, primarily because the egg for the next cycle reaches maximum sensitivity during the 10-day period. The application of this guideline within the radiology department has always proven difficult.

It is now the general belief that postponement of abdominal x-ray examinations is not necessary when the physician requesting the examination has considered the entire clinical state of the patient, including the possibility of pregnancy. The potential pregnancy status of all female patients of childbearing age should always be determined; in the event of known pregnancy, steps should be taken to minimize exposure to the fetus. One way to ensure against irradiating a woman in the early stages of pregnancy is to institute elective scheduling for nonemergency procedures. In many departments, female patients of childbearing ages are asked to provide the date of their last menstrual period (LMP). If there is a concern about a possible pregnancy, the patient's exam may be rescheduled. If a radiologic exam on a pregnant patient is deemed necessary, a diagnostic radiological physicist should perform calculations to estimate the actual fetal dose.

REPEAT RADIOGRAPHS

Repeat radiographs, which range from approximately 5–15%, result in additional patient exposure. Repeat examinations resulting from carelessness or poor radiographer judgment must be eliminated. The radiographer should select correct radiographic techniques and exposure factors that ensure high-quality radiographs.

Causes of repeat radiographs also include dirty screens, incorrectly loaded cassettes, light leaks, chemical fog, processor artifacts, incorrect projections, positioning errors, grid errors, and multiple exposures.

FLUOROSCOPIC PROCEDURES

Fluoroscopy produces the greatest patient radiation exposure in diagnostic radiology. Because x-ray exposures produce cumulative effects, the physician should evaluate the necessity of the exam. If the physician judges the exam necessary, precautions must be taken to minimize patient dose.

Image Intensification Fluoroscopy

This system converts the x-ray into an amplified visible light pattern. Image brightness increases approximately 7,000–20,000 times with **image intensification fluoroscopy**, as compared to conventional fluoroscopic systems. With the use of image intensified fluoroscopy, the radiologist does not need to go through dark adaptation, as was necessary with conventional fluoroscopy. This increase in image brightness results in the use of less mA (approximately 1.5–2 mA for image intensification systems, as compared to 3–5 mA for conventional fluoroscopy). The consequent decrease in exposure rate results in a reduction in dose for the patient.

Intermittent Fluoroscopy   The radiologist should use **intermittent fluoroscopy** to decrease patient exposure and prolong tube life. This means the radiologist should periodically activate the fluoroscopic tube, rather than having the tube continuously activated.

Limitation of Field Size   Limitation of field size is accomplished by placing lead collimating shutters between the fluoroscopic tube and the patient. The fluoroscopic beam must be restricted to the smallest field that includes the area of interest, which reduces exposure to both patient and personnel. The radiologist should collimate to only the area of interest. Federal law prohibits the useful beam at the image receptor from exceeding the visible image area by more than 3% of the source-image receptor distance (SID).

Exposure Factors   The recommended operating factors are 90–100 kVp, 2–3 mA, and 2.5 mm Al equivalent filter for image intensified fluoroscopy. According to federal law, the source-tabletop distance must be at least 15 in. (38 cm) with stationary and 12 in. (30 cm) with mobile fluoroscopic equipment. Fluoroscopic exposure factors for pediatric patients necessitate a decrease in kVp by as much as 25%. The chosen kVp depends on thickness of part, the same as it does during conventional radiography.

A **cumulative timing device** must be furnished and used with all fluoroscopic units. This device is provided to preset the on-time of the fluoroscopic tube for a cumulative total of no more than five minutes. An audible signal will sound when five minutes has accumulated, and will continue to sound until the timer is reset to five minutes.

According to federal code, the exposure rate at the tabletop must be no greater than 10 R/min for fluoroscopic equipment with intensified fluoroscopic units and no greater than 5 R/min without intensified fluoroscopic units.

KEY CONCEPTS

- It is important to keep the patient immobilized to avoid artifact in the x-ray and to avoid repeat exposures.
- Beam limiting apparatus serve to control the direction of the beam to specific areas of the body. Collimators are the best device for this purpose.
- X-ray beam filtration reduces patient exposure by use of a filter to absorb low energy photons.
- It is important to use gonadal shielding to protect the patient's reproductive organs from radiation exposure. There are several

varieties of shields used: flat contact shields, shadow shields, and shaped contact shields.

- Use of correct exposure factors limits the need for repeat exposures; factors to consider are high kVp and low mAs and high speed intensifying screens.
- Use of high speed intensifying screens converts x-ray energy into visible light thus reducing the exposure of the patient to radiation.
- Reducing the number of repeat radiographs reduces the radiation exposure of both the patient and the radiographer.
- Radiation exposure during flouroscopic procedures can be limited by using intermittent flouroscopy and reducing the size of the exposed field.

SECTION REVIEW

1. How tall must primary protective barriers be?
   a. 3 feet
   b. 4 feet
   c. 7 feet
   d. 10 feet

2. Leakage radiation from the x-ray tube housing shall not exceed _____ at a distance of 1 meter from the tube.
   a. 1 mR/hr
   b. 10 mR/hr
   c. 100 mR/hr
   d. 1,000 mR/hr

3. The minimum lead equivalency of a lead apron must be at least
   a. 0.12 mm
   b. 0.25 mm
   c. 0.5 mm
   d. 1 mm

4. How many rems whole body cumulative exposure would a 45-year-old radiographer be allowed to receive?
   a. 15
   b. 45
   c. 35
   d. 25

5. A protective lead curtain that is at least _____ Pb equivalent must be positioned between the patient and the fluoroscopy operator.
   a. 0.025 mm
   b. 0.25 mm
   c. 2.5 mm
   d. 25 mm

6. The function of a filter is to remove which of the following from the x-ray beam?
    a. short wavelength radiation
    b. long wavelength radiation
    c. secondary radiation
    d. scattered radiation

7. Which of the following is the best type of gonadal shielding to use during a sterile field procedure?
    a. flat contact shields
    b. shadow shields
    c. shaped contact shields
    d. lead sheet

8. A fluoroscope must be equipped with a cumulative timing device which times the radiation exposure and sounds an audible alarm after the fluoroscope has been energized for
    a. 1 minute
    b. 2 minutes
    c. 3 minutes
    d. 5 minutes

9. Which of the following is not a type of beam limitation device?
    a. collimator
    b. cone
    c. filter
    d. aperture diaphragm

10. The minimum source to tabletop distance permitted in mobile fluoroscopy is
    a. 4 inches
    b. 9 inches
    c. 12 inches
    d. 15 inches

CASE STUDY 1

You are about to perform a mobile x-ray exam on your patient. Discuss how you should utilize the three cardinal principles of radiation protection for you and your patient.

CASE STUDY 2

You are about to x-ray a patient who is exhibiting voluntary motion. Discuss what steps you would take to minimize this motion. Compare this with involuntary motion.

Bibliography

Bushberg, J., Seibert, J., Leidholdt, E., & Boone, J. (1994). *The essentials physics of medical imaging.* Baltimore: Williams & Wilkins.

Bushong, S. (1997). *Radiologic science for technologists* (6th ed.). St. Louis, MO: C.V. Mosby.

Carlton, R., & Adler, A. (2001). *Principles of radiographic imaging: An art and science* (3rd ed.). Albany, NY: Delmar/Thomson Learning.

Dowd, S., & Tilson, E. (1999). *Practical radiation protection and applied radiobiology* (2nd ed.). Philadelphia: Saunders.

Fong, E., Scott, A., Ferris, E., & Skelley, E. (1993). *Body structures and functions* (8th wd.). Albany, NY: Delmar.

Gurley, L., & Callaway, W. (1992). *Introduction to radiologic technology* (3rd wd.) St. Louis, MO: C.V. Mosby.

Hendee, W., & Ritenour, R. (1992). *Medical imaging physics* (3rd Ed.). St. Louis: C.V Mobsy.

National Council on Radiation Protection and Measurements, Bethesda, Maryland.

Scanlon, V., & Saunder, T. (1991). *Essentials of anatomy and physiology*, Philadelphia, PA: F.A. Davis.

Seeram, E. (1997). *Radiation protection.* Philadelphia/New York: Lipincott.

Selman, J. (1985). *The fundamentals of X-ray and radium physics* (7th ed.). Springfield, IL: Thomas.

Statkiewicz-Sherer, M., Visconti, P., & Ritenour, E. (1993). *Radiation protection in medical radiography* (2nd wd.). St. Louis, MO: C.V. Mosby,.

Thompson, M., Hattaway, M., Hall, J., & Dowd, S. (1994). *Principles of imaging science and protection*, Philadelphia: Saunders.

Tortora, G., & Grabowski, S. (1993). *Principles of anatomy and physiology*, New York, NY: Harper Collins.

Travis, E. (1989). *Primer of medical radiobiology* (2nd ed.). Chicago: YearBook Medical Publishers.

VandeGraaff, K., & Fox, S. (1989). *Concepts of human anatomy and physiology* (2nd ed.). Columbus, OH: Wm. C. Brown Publishers.

Glossary

A

Aberration Imperfection.

Absolute risk model (1) Estimates a continual increase in risk, independent of the age-specific cancer risk at time of exposure; also known as the additive risk model. (2) number of cases per 10^6 persons per rad per year.

Acentric On the outside; the periphery.

Acute Rapid, severe.

Added filtration Limiting the x-ray beam by the use of a piece of aluminum or aluminum equivalent outside the glass window of the housing tube.

Agreement states Those states that have agreements with the Nuclear Regulatory Commission to take responsibility to enforce radiation protection guidelines through the states department of health.

ALARA As low as reasonably achievable.

Alopecia Hair loss.

Amino acid An organic compound which is the building block of proteins, and the end product of protein digestion.

Anabolism The construction phase of metabolism, when a cell takes the substances from blood that are necessary for repair and growth, and converts them into cytoplasm. The opposite of catabolism.

Anaphase A stage in mitosis and meiosis between metaphase and telophase in which chromatids migrate toward opposite poles of the cell.

Anemia Reduction in red blood cell counts.

Ankylosing spondylitis Immobility of the vertebrae.

Anomaly Departure from normal.

Aperture diaphragm A piece of flat lead with a hole in the center. This equipment is attached to the tube to confine the x-ray beam to the area of the hole. All areas surrounding the hole will remain unexposed.

Atrophy Shrinking.

Autosomes Any chromosome that is other than the sex (X and Y) chromosomes.

B

Beam limitation device Equipment that reduces the beam to only those areas in need of exposure; all other areas will not be exposed to the beam.

BEIR Committee on the Biological Effects of Ionizing Radiation.

Benign Nonprogressive.

Bone marrow dose A measure of the radiation that has been absorbed into the patient's bone marrow.

C

Carcinogenic Cancer causing.

Carcinoma A growth or tumor.

Catabolism The destructive phase of metabolism, in which complex substances are changed into simpler substances. The opposite of anabolism.

Centromere The constricted area of the chromosome that separates the chromosome into two arms.

Chromatid The halves into which the chromosome is longitudinally divided, which are held together by the centromere and move to opposite poles of a dividing cell during anaphase.

Chromatin A material in the nucleus which contains genetic information. It is DNA which is joined to a protein structure base.

Chromosome The linear thread of a cell nucleus. They contain DNA, which makes up genes, our hereditary blueprint.

Chronic Slow, progressive.

Cones A circular metal structure attached to the x-ray tube housing to restrict the x-ray beam to a predetermined size.

Controlled area An area occupied by radiation personnel.

Crypts of Lieberkuhn Radiosensitive cells precursor to the population of villi cells.

Cumulative timing device A device that presets the on time for the tube to only five minute increments.

Cytopenia Depression of all blood cell counts.

D

Deadman type Exposure control switch that is either a foot pedal or a hand switch.

Deletion A chromosomal effect that causes a loss of genetic material.

Deoxyribonucleic acid (DNA) A polymer composed of deoxyribonucleotides. Arranged in a double helix, it is present in chromosomes in the cell's nucleus, and is the carrier of genetic information.

Dermis Middle layer of the skin.

Desquamation Peeling skin.

Dicentric A chromosome which has two centers or two centromeres.

Diploid Possessing two sets of chromosomes, in reference to somatic cells, which have two times the number of chromosomes present in the egg or sperm. Referred to as 2n; in humans, the 2n or diploid number = 46.

Direct effect A result of ionization and excitation, an interaction that happens directly on a critical biologic macromolecule.

Dose Amount of radiation exposure.

Dose-response relationship (curve) A graphical representation of observed effects (response) compared with radiation dose.

Dosimetry Measurement of ionizing radiation doses to personnel.

Doubling dose The dose of radiation required per generation to double the spontaneous mutation rate.

Duplication A chromosome mutation in which either one or both segments of a chromosome join to another chromosome.

E

Early effect of radiation The response of human cells exposed to radiation within minutes, days or weeks of exposure.

Edema Swelling.

Effective dose-equivalent limit The lowest does of radiation that will maintain health with no ill effects.

Effectiveness A graphical representation of observed effects compared with radiation dose.

Entrance skin exposure (ESE) A measure of the radiation to the patient's skin at the skin entrance surface; also known as the skin dose.

Enzyme A complex organic protein which accelerates chemical reactions.

Epidermis Outer layer of the skin

Epilation Hair loss.

Erythema Reddening of skin.

Erythroblasts Precursors for red blood cells.

Excess risk The number of excess cases of cancer observed compared with expected spontaneous occurrence.

F

Fibrosis Abnormal formation of fibrous tissue.

Film badge A type of dosimeter consisting of radiation dosimetry film to determine the amount of exposure personnel have received.

Flat contact shield Rubberized lead strips that are placed over areas of the body to protect them from exposure.

Follicle Sac or cavity.

Follicular Cavity.

Fractionation The splitting of radiation into smaller amounts over a period of time.

Free radical An atom which has an unpaired electron making it highly reactive. It is produced as a result of radiolysis of water.

G

G_1 The gap or growth period between telophase and the start of DNA synthesis when DNA is not replicating.

G_2 The gap or growth period following the replication of DNA and prior to mitosis.

Gamete The mature male (spermatozoon) or female (ovum) reproductive cell.

Gene The basic unit of heredity which has a specific location on a chromosome.

Genetically significant dose (GSD) An average calculated from the gonadal dose received by the entire population and used to determine the genetic influence of low dose to the whole population.

Gonad shielding Protection of the reproductive organs from radiation exposure.

Gonadal dose A measure of the radiation to the patient at the site of the patient's gonads.

Granulocytes Red blood cells with a life cycle of one day.

H

Half-value layer (HVL) The thickness of the material which will reduce the x-ray intensity to half its original value.

Haploid Having half the diploid number of chromosomes found in somatic cells. Referred to as n; in humans, the n or haploid number = 23.

HeLa Letters which represent the first two letters of the patient's first and last names in an experiment conducted by Puck using uterine cervix cells to produce cell cultures.

Hemopoietic Pertaining to the development of blood cells.

Hypoxic Low levels of oxygen.

I

Image intensification flouroscopy A procedure used to increase the brightness of an image with a decreased exposure time.

Indirect effect A cell interaction which occurs if the initial ionizing incident takes place on a distant noncritical molecule which then transfers the ionization of energy to another molecule.

Inflammation Redness and swelling at site of exposure.

Inherent filtration Limiting the x-ray beam by the use of a glass window in the tube and cooling oil surrounding the tube housing.

Intensifying screen A device that serves to accelerate the action of x-rays by converting x-ray energy into visible light.

Intermittent fluoroscopy The procedure of periodically activating the flouroscopic tube rather than having the tube continuously activated; this reduces patient exposure and prolongs the life of the tube.

Interphase The period between cell divisions, known as the resting stage, when DNA is being synthesized. (Also known as S phase, S = synthesis.)

Interphase death Cell death occurring before mitosis.

Inverse square law The intensity of radiation at a given distance is inversely proportional to the square of the distance of the object from the source.

Involuntary motion Movement by the patient that is beyond his control.

Ionization chamber A tube containing a positive and negative electrode that are charged before use. One electrode is stationary, the other is moving. Exposure to ionization is determined by measurement of movement of the moving electrode.

J

Joint Commission on the Accreditation of Healthcare Organizations (JCAHO) The accreditating body for radiographic facilities.

K

Karyotype Chromosome map.

L

Late effect of radiation The response of human cells exposed to radiation months to years after exposure.

Latent The second stage in the response to radiation exposure in which changes are taking place within the body system that may either result in death or recovery.

Law of Bergonie and Tribondeau Law which states that ionizing radiation is more effective against cells which are highly mitotic, immature, and have a long dividing future; named for the two experimenters who made this determination.

LD50/30 The survival time of a specific group; the lethal dose to kill 50% of a population in 30 days.

LD50/60 The survival time of a specific group; the lethal dose to kill 50% of a population in 60 days.

Lead equivalent The amount of material that is needed to meet the same requirements as a lead barrier.

Lesion Open wound.

Leukemia Cancer of blood forming cells in bone marrow.

Linear dose-response curve Graphical representation of relationship between radiation dose and observed response, in which any dose may have a potential effect, and there is a direction relationship between radiation dose and observed effect.

Linear energy transfer (LET) A measure of the rate at which energy is deposited from ionizing radiation to soft tissue.

Linear quadratic dose-response curve Graphical representation of relationship between radiation dose and observed response, in which the curve is linear or proportional at low doses, and becomes curvilinear at higher doses. This type of curve has no threshold.

Loci Spot, place of origin.

Lymphoid Lymph tissue.

M

Macromolecule A large molecule, for example, proteins, polymers, nucleic acids, and polysaccharides.

Malignant Progressive; threatening.

Manifest The third stage in the response to radiation exposure in which body systems show signs and symptoms of exposure.

Maturation depletion Reduction in the number of mature sperm.

Megakaryocytes Precursors for platelets.

Meiosis Cell division of germ cells, which consists of two cell divisions but only one replication of DNA. This results in each daughter cell containing one-half the number of chromosomes that are characteristic of the somatic cells of that species.

Meningitis Inflammation of the membranes of the spinal cord and brain.

Messenger RNA (m-RNA) RNA that binds amino acids to ribosomes during protein synthesis.

Metaphase The stage of mitosis where chromosomes are arranged.

Mitosis Type of cell division involving somatic cells in which a parent cell divides to create two daughter cells that contain the same chromosome number and DNA content as the parent. A continuous process having four phases: prophase, metaphase, anaphase, and telophase.

Mutagenesis The causing of genetic mutation by radiation.

Mutation A structural change or transformation of a chromosome which can be transmitted to offspring.

Myelocytes Precursors for white blood cells.

Myeloid Marrow.

N

Necrosis Tissue death.

Neoplasm Tumor.

Neuroblasts Embryonic nerve cells.

Nonstochastic Deterministic.

Nonthreshold Any dose received, regardless of size, which will produce a response.

Nuclear membrane Also referred to as the nuclear envelope; a two-layered membrane which surrounds the cell nucleus.

Nucleolus Spherical body in the cell nucleus that holds nuclear RNA. On the equatorial cell plane prior to separation, follows prophase and precedes anaphase.

O

Oogonia Reproductive cells of the female.

Organism Any living entity; may be unicellular or multicellular.

Osteosarcoma Bone cancer.

Oxygen effect Name given to cellular response to radiation when oxygen is present.

P

Papillary Nipple-like protrusion.

Parenchymal Essential life-sustaining cells.

Personnel dosimeters Devices used to measure radiation doses.

Pocket dosimeter A type of dosimeter that uses an ionization chamber to determine the level of exposure by personnel.

Point mutation A mutation which occurs as a result from a change of a single DNA base pair, created by one nucleotide being exchanged for another.

Polymer A molecule created by combining two or more of the same molecules.

Primary protective barrier A fixed barrier that is located perpendicular to the line of travel of the primary x-ray beam.

Prodromal The first stage in the response to radiation exposure; nausea, vomiting, and diarrhea usually occur in this stage of exposure.

Progeny Offspring.

Prophase The first stage of mitosis or meiosis, when chromosomes become visible.

Protective tube housing The lead lined metal covering of the x-ray beam that serves to reduce leakage radiation.

Protoplasm A colloidal structure of organic and inorganic materials and water which form the living cell.

R

Rad The unit of radiation absorbed dose.

Radiation cataractogenesis Formation of cataracts caused by exposure to radiation.

Radiation protection Methods used to limit exposure to radiation.

Radioactivity The capability of a material to give off rays or particles from its nucleus.

Radiobiology Division of biology concerned with effects of ionizing radiation on living things.

Radiocarcinogenesis Radiation producing cancer.

Radiolysis Breakdown of water using radiation.

Radioresistant Having no reaction or ill effects of exposure to radiation.

Radiosensitivity The amount of reaction or response of a cell to radiation.

Radium Radiogenic substance.

Radon Radiogenic gas.

Relative biologic effectiveness (RBE) A comparison of how effective types of radiation are compared with x- and gamma-rays.

Relative risk model (1) Relates age at the time of radiation exposure to cancer risk estimate; also known as the multiplicative risk model. (2) The ratio of cancer incidence in an exposed population to that of an unexposed population.

Rem The unit of dose equivalent or occupational exposure.

Reproductive failure Cell which is unable to continue repeated divisions after being irradiated.

Ribonucleic acid (RNA) Nucleic acid which controls protein synthesis. Differs from DNA by having ribose as its sugar and the base uracil instead of thymine. Types include messenger, transfer, and ribosomal RNA.

Ribosomal RNA RNA that exists in ribosomes and assists in protein synthesis.

Ring Mutation of chromosome causing it to become ring-shaped.

Roentgen (R) A unit of radiation exposure descriptive of x- or gamma-radiation, the quantity of which would produce a charge of one electrostatic unit of electricity.

S

Scattered radiation Radiation that is dissipated away from the point of origin.

Sebaceous Oily secretion.

Secondary protective barrier A fixed barrier that is located parallel to the line of travel of the primary x-ray beam.

SED50 Radiation dose necessary to affect 50% of a population.

Shadow shield A radiopaque material that is suspended from the tube housing which casts a shadow over the area that should not be exposed.

Shaped contact shield Lead devices that are shaped to fit over anatomical areas of the body to protect them from radiation exposure.

Sigmoid An S-shaped type of dose-response relationship.

Skin dose A measure of the radiation to the patient's skin at the skin entrance surface; also known as the entrance skin exposure (ESE).

Skin erythema dose (SED) A measure of the amount of radiation a person received.

Somatic Nonreproductive cells.

Source-image receptor distance (SID) The area from the point of contact on the patient to the tube.

Spermatogonia Reproductive cells of the male.

S-phase Period of synthesis or replication, the phase of the cell cycle after G1 and prior to G2.

Stem cell Immature cells.

Stochastic Occurring randomly in nature.

Stroma Supportive tissue of an organism.

Subcutaneous Inner layer of skin; the fatty layer.

Syndrome The relationship of signs and symptoms to a specific disease or trauma.

System A group of cells which perform a particular function.

T

Telophase The fourth or final stage of mitosis or meiosis, during which there is reconstruction of the nuclear membrane, and cell cytoplasm divides, giving birth to two daughter cells.

Thermoluminescent dosimeters (TLD) A type of dosimeter containing lithium flouride or calcium flouride crystals to calculate the amount of personnel exposure.

Threshold The point where a stimulus starts to produce an effect.

Threshold dose The dose at which symptoms will occur.

Time of occupancy (T) The amount of time a hospital area is occupied by people.

Total filtration The maximum amount of limitation of the x-ray beam through the use of both added and inherent filtration methods.

Transfer RNA (t-RNA) RNA that carries amino acids to ribosomes for assisting in protein synthesis.

Translocation Altering of a chromosome either by a portion of it transferring to another chromosome or to another section of the same chromosome.

Turner's syndrome An endocrine disorder caused by the failure of the ovaries to respond to pituitary hormone stimulation.

U

Uncontrolled area An area occupied by non-radiation personnel.

Use (U) The percentage of time in which the x-ray beam is energized and directed toward a particular wall.

Useful beam The primary x-ray beam.

V

Variable-aperture collimator A pair of upper and lower level lead shutters at right angles to each other. They can be adjusted to limit the field size the x-ray beam will expose.

Vasculitis Inflammation of blood vessels.

Voluntary motion Movement controlled by the patient.

W

Workload (W) The amount of activity of the x-ray machinery.

Z

Zygote Fertilized egg.

Index

Notes

Notes

Notes

Notes